CHAPTER 1: INTRODUCTION TO GLIOBLASTOMA

Definition and Classification of Glioblastoma

Glioblastoma (GBM) stands as one of the most aggressive and lethal primary brain tumors. Its classification and definition have evolved over time, reflecting advances in understanding its biological behavior and molecular characteristics. In this discourse, we delve into the intricate details of defining and classifying GBM, exploring its historical context, morphological features, and molecular subtypes.

At its core, Glioblastoma represents a type of glioma, arising from glial cells, the supportive cells of the central nervous system (CNS). Specifically, it originates from astrocytes, a type of glial cell responsible for maintaining the structural integrity of the brain and supporting neuronal function. Glioblastoma is characterized by its rapid growth, diffuse infiltration into surrounding brain tissue, and resistance to conventional therapies.

Historical Context: The history of GBM classification dates back to the early 20th century when pioneering neurosurgeons and neuropathologists first described tumors of the brain. The term "glioblastoma" was coined by German neurologist Wilhelm Schultze in 1895, who observed its highly malignant nature under the microscope. Over the decades, advancements in neuroimaging, histopathology, and molecular biology have reshaped our understanding of GBM, leading to refined classification schemes.

Morphological Features: Traditionally, GBMs were classified based on their histological characteristics, primarily observed through microscopic examination of tissue samples obtained via biopsy or surgical resection. These tumors exhibit marked cellular and nuclear pleomorphism, high mitotic activity, microvascular proliferation, and necrosis. The presence of these features distinguishes GBM from lower-grade gliomas and informs clinical management and prognosis.

World Health Organization (WHO) Classification: The WHO classification system serves as the cornerstone for categorizing central nervous system tumors, including GBM. The most recent iteration, WHO Classification of Tumours of the Central Nervous System, 5th edition (2021), provides a comprehensive framework for diagnosing and grading gliomas based on histological and molecular criteria. According to WHO criteria, GBM is classified as a grade IV astrocytoma, reflecting its highest degree of malignancy.

Molecular Subtypes: In recent years, molecular profiling has emerged as a powerful tool for subclassifying GBM and guiding personalized treatment strategies. Through genome-wide analyses, researchers have identified distinct molecular subtypes of GBM characterized by specific genetic alterations and signaling pathways. These subtypes include classical, mesenchymal, proneural, and neural, each with unique biological behaviors and therapeutic vulnerabilities.

Clinical Implications: Accurate classification of GBM is paramount for guiding treatment decisions and predicting patient outcomes. Histological and molecular features not only inform prognosis but also influence therapeutic strategies, such as the use of targeted agents and immunotherapy. Furthermore, molecular subtyping holds promise for identifying novel therapeutic targets and developing more effective treatment regimens tailored to individual patients.

Conclusion: In summary, Glioblastoma represents a formidable challenge in neuro-oncology, characterized by its aggressive nature and dismal prognosis. Defining and classifying GBM involves a multidimensional approach, integrating histological, molecular, and clinical criteria. By elucidating its morphological and molecular features, we can refine our understanding of GBM pathogenesis and pave the way for innovative therapeutic interventions aimed at improving patient outcomes.

Epidemiology of Glioblastoma: Understanding the Burden and Trends

Glioblastoma (GBM) poses a significant public health challenge, with its aggressive nature and poor prognosis imposing a substantial burden on individuals, families, and healthcare systems worldwide. In this exploration of GBM epidemiology, we delve into its incidence, prevalence, risk factors, geographic variations, and temporal trends, seeking to unravel the complex interplay of factors that contribute to the occurrence and distribution of this devastating disease.

Incidence and Prevalence: Glioblastoma represents the most common primary malignant brain tumor in adults, comprising approximately 15-20% of all primary brain tumors and 50-60% of all gliomas. Its annual incidence varies geographically, with higher rates reported in developed countries compared to developing nations. In the United States, the age-adjusted incidence rate of GBM is estimated to be around 3-4 cases per 100,000 population per year.

Age and Gender Distribution: GBM predominantly affects adults, with peak incidence occurring in the sixth and seventh decades of life. While rare in children and young adults, GBM incidence increases with advancing age, reflecting age-related changes in cellular physiology and DNA repair mechanisms. Additionally, GBM exhibits a slight male predominance, with men being slightly more susceptible to the disease than women.

Geographic and Racial Disparities: Studies have identified geographic and racial disparities in GBM incidence and survival, with higher rates observed in certain regions and populations. For instance, Caucasian individuals have a higher incidence of GBM compared to African American, Hispanic, and Asian/Pacific Islander populations. Geographic variations in GBM incidence may be attributed to differences in environmental exposures, genetic predisposition, healthcare access, and diagnostic practices.

Environmental and Occupational Risk Factors: While the precise etiology of GBM remains elusive, several environmental and occupational factors have been implicated in its pathogenesis. Exposure to ionizing radiation, such as therapeutic radiation for previous cancers or occupational radiation exposure, is a well-established risk factor for GBM development. Other potential risk factors include exposure to certain chemical agents, such as pesticides, solvents, and industrial pollutants, although the evidence remains inconclusive.

Genetic and Familial Factors: A small proportion of GBM cases are associated with hereditary cancer syndromes, such as neurofibromatosis type 1 (NF1), Li-Fraumeni syndrome, and Turcot syndrome. Additionally, emerging evidence suggests that germline mutations in genes involved in DNA repair pathways, such as BRCA1 and BRCA2, may confer an increased risk of developing GBM. However, the majority of GBM cases are sporadic, with no identifiable genetic predisposition.

Temporal Trends: Over the past few decades, there has been growing concern regarding the rising incidence of GBM and other primary brain tumors. While improvements in diagnostic techniques and population-based cancer registries may partly account for the observed increase, some studies suggest a true rise in incidence, possibly linked to changes in environmental exposures, lifestyle factors, or other yet unidentified risk factors.

Conclusion: In conclusion, the epidemiology of Glioblastoma is complex and multifaceted, shaped by a myriad of genetic, environmental, and lifestyle factors. While advances in research have expanded our understanding of GBM etiology and risk factors, many questions remain unanswered. Continued efforts to elucidate the underlying mechanisms driving GBM development and progression are crucial for informing preventive strategies, early detection methods, and targeted interventions aimed at reducing the burden of this devastating disease on individuals and society.

Etiology and Risk Factors of Glioblastoma: Unraveling the Complex Puzzle

Glioblastoma (GBM) is a devastating disease characterized by its aggressive growth and poor prognosis. Understanding the etiology and risk factors underlying GBM development is essential for elucidating its pathogenesis, informing preventive strategies, and guiding targeted interventions. In this exploration, we delve into the multifaceted etiological factors and potential risk determinants implicated in the onset and progression of GBM.

Genetic Alterations and Molecular Pathways: At the core of GBM etiology lie complex genetic alterations and dysregulated molecular pathways that drive tumorigenesis and disease progression. Advances in genomic sequencing technologies have revealed recurrent genetic mutations and chromosomal aberrations in GBM, including alterations in tumor suppressor genes (e.g., TP53, PTEN), oncogenes (e.g., EGFR, IDH1), and DNA repair genes (e.g., MGMT). Dysregulation of signaling pathways, such as the phosphatidylinositol 3-kinase (PI3K)/Akt/mTOR pathway and the mitogen-activated protein kinase (MAPK) pathway, further contribute to the malignant phenotype of GBM.

Environmental Exposures: Exposure to environmental carcinogens and toxicants has been implicated as potential risk factors for GBM development. Ionizing radiation, such as therapeutic radiation for previous cancers or occupational radiation exposure, is a well-established risk factor for GBM, leading to DNA damage and genomic instability. Additionally, certain chemical agents, including pesticides, solvents, and industrial pollutants, have been associated with an increased risk of GBM, although the evidence remains inconclusive and requires further investigation.

Inherited Predisposition: While the majority of GBM cases are sporadic, a small proportion are associated with hereditary cancer syndromes and germline mutations in predisposing genes. Neurofibromatosis type 1 (NF1), Li-Fraumeni syndrome, and Turcot syndrome are among the hereditary conditions linked to an elevated risk of developing GBM. Additionally, germline mutations in genes involved in DNA repair pathways, such as BRCA1 and BRCA2, may confer an increased susceptibility to GBM, highlighting the role of inherited genetic factors in disease susceptibility.

Age and Gender: GBM incidence increases with advancing age, with peak occurrence in the sixth and seventh decades of life. Age-related changes in cellular physiology, DNA repair mechanisms, and cumulative exposure to environmental factors may contribute to the higher susceptibility of older individuals to GBM. Furthermore, GBM exhibits a slight male predominance, with men being slightly more susceptible to the disease than women, although the underlying reasons for this gender disparity remain poorly understood.

Viral Infections: Emerging evidence suggests a potential role of viral infections in GBM pathogenesis, although the exact mechanisms remain elusive. Human cytomegalovirus (HCMV) and simian virus 40 (SV40) are among the viruses implicated in GBM, with studies reporting their presence in tumor tissues and association with disease progression. However, the causal relationship between viral infections and GBM development requires further investigation to elucidate the underlying mechanisms and potential therapeutic implications.

Conclusion: In conclusion, the etiology of Glioblastoma is multifactorial, involving a complex interplay of genetic, environmental, and lifestyle factors. Genetic alterations and dysregulated molecular pathways drive tumorigenesis and disease progression, while environmental exposures, inherited predisposition, age, gender, and viral infections contribute to individual susceptibility to GBM. Continued research efforts aimed at unraveling the intricate mechanisms underlying GBM etiology are crucial for developing preventive strategies, identifying novel therapeutic targets, and improving patient outcomes in the battle against this devastating disease.

Pathophysiology of Glioblastoma: Unraveling the Molecular Complexity

Glioblastoma (GBM) is characterized by its aggressive growth, diffuse infiltration into surrounding brain tissue, and resistance to conventional therapies. Understanding the underlying pathophysiology of GBM is essential for elucidating its biological behavior, guiding treatment strategies, and identifying novel therapeutic targets. In this exploration, we delve into the intricate molecular mechanisms driving GBM pathogenesis, highlighting key signaling pathways, cellular interactions, and microenvironmental factors involved in disease progression.

Genetic Alterations: GBM is characterized by extensive genetic alterations that disrupt cellular homeostasis and drive oncogenesis. Key genetic mutations implicated in GBM pathophysiology include alterations in tumor suppressor genes (e.g., TP53, PTEN), oncogenes (e.g., EGFR, PDGFRA), and DNA repair genes (e.g., MGMT). These mutations result in dysregulated cell cycle control, aberrant proliferation, evasion of apoptosis, and genomic instability, contributing to the malignant phenotype of GBM.

Molecular Signaling Pathways: Dysregulated molecular

signaling pathways play a pivotal role in GBM pathophysiology, driving tumorigenesis and disease progression. The phosphatidylinositol 3-kinase (PI3K)/Akt/mTOR pathway and the mitogen-activated protein kinase (MAPK) pathway are among the key signaling cascades implicated in GBM. Activation of these pathways promotes cell survival, proliferation, invasion, and angiogenesis, while inhibiting apoptosis and immune responses, thereby fueling tumor growth and metastasis.

Tumor Microenvironment: The tumor microenvironment plays a critical role in GBM pathophysiology, shaping tumor growth, invasion, and therapeutic response. GBM is characterized by a complex interplay between tumor cells, stromal cells, immune cells, and extracellular matrix components. Tumor-associated microglia/macrophages (TAMs), cancer-associated fibroblasts (CAFs), and endothelial cells contribute to tumor growth and angiogenesis, while infiltrating immune cells modulate the anti-tumor immune response and promote immune evasion.

Angiogenesis: Angiogenesis, the process of new blood vessel formation, is a hallmark of GBM pathophysiology and is crucial for tumor growth and progression. Hypoxia-induced upregulation of pro-angiogenic factors, such as vascular endothelial growth factor (VEGF) and hypoxia-inducible factor 1-alpha (HIF-1α), promotes the formation of abnormal and leaky blood vessels within the tumor microenvironment. Disruption of the blood-brain barrier further facilitates tumor invasion and metastasis, while limiting the delivery of therapeutic agents to tumor cells.

Immune Evasion Mechanisms: GBM employs various immune evasion mechanisms to evade detection and destruction by the host immune system. Tumor cells express immune checkpoint molecules, such as programmed cell death ligand 1 (PD-L1) and cytotoxic T-lymphocyte-associated protein 4 (CTLA-4), which suppress T-cell activation and promote immune tolerance. Additionally, GBM cells release immunosuppressive cytokines and recruit regulatory T cells (Tregs) and myeloid-derived suppressor cells (MDSCs) to inhibit anti-tumor immune responses and promote tumor immune escape.

Metabolic Reprogramming: Metabolic reprogramming is a hallmark of cancer, including GBM, enabling tumor cells to adapt to the nutrient-deprived and hypoxic tumor microenvironment. GBM cells exhibit enhanced glycolysis and lactate production, even in the presence of oxygen (aerobic glycolysis), a phenomenon known as the Warburg effect. Alterations in mitochondrial metabolism, lipid metabolism, and amino acid metabolism further support tumor growth and survival in the nutrient-poor tumor microenvironment.

Conclusion: In conclusion, the pathophysiology of Glioblastoma is characterized by a complex interplay of genetic alterations, dysregulated molecular signaling pathways, tumor microenvironment interactions, angiogenesis, immune evasion mechanisms, and metabolic reprogramming. Elucidating the molecular complexity of GBM is essential for developing targeted therapeutic strategies aimed at disrupting key signaling pathways, modulating the tumor microenvironment, and overcoming treatment resistance in the quest for more effective treatments and improved outcomes for patients with this devastating disease.

CHAPTER 2: ANATOMY OF THE BRAIN

Overview of Brain Structure: Understanding the Architectural Complexity

The human brain stands as one of the most intricate and sophisticated organs in the body, orchestrating a multitude of complex functions that underpin cognition, behavior, and emotion. In this exploration of brain structure, we embark on a journey through its anatomical organization, highlighting key regions, structures, and functional networks that contribute to its remarkable capabilities.

The Central Nervous System (CNS): The brain is the central hub of the nervous system, along with the spinal cord, comprising the central nervous system (CNS). Encased within the protective confines of the skull, the brain serves as the command center for the body, integrating sensory information, coordinating motor responses, and regulating vital physiological processes.

Major Divisions of the Brain: The human brain can be broadly divided into three major regions: the forebrain, midbrain, and hindbrain. Each region plays distinct roles in sensory processing, motor control, and higher cognitive functions.

Forebrain: The forebrain is the largest and most complex region of the brain, encompassing the cerebral hemispheres, thalamus, and hypothalamus. The cerebral hemispheres, comprising the left and right cerebral cortices, are responsible for higher-order functions such as perception, cognition, language, and emotion. The thalamus serves as a relay station for sensory information, transmitting signals to the cerebral cortex for further processing. The hypothalamus plays a critical role in regulating autonomic functions, hormone secretion, and homeostatic mechanisms.

Midbrain: The midbrain, situated between the forebrain and hindbrain, contains several important structures involved in sensory processing, motor coordination, and arousal. The tectum, comprising the superior and inferior colliculi, plays a key role in visual and auditory reflexes. The tegmentum houses the substantia nigra, a dopaminergic nucleus implicated in motor control and reward processing.

Hindbrain: The hindbrain, located posterior to the midbrain, consists of the cerebellum, pons, and medulla oblongata. The cerebellum, often referred to as the "little brain," is essential for coordinating movement, maintaining balance, and motor learning. The pons serves as a relay center, connecting the cerebellum to the cerebral cortex and facilitating communication between different regions of the brain. The medulla oblongata controls vital autonomic functions such as respiration, heart rate, and blood pressure.

Cerebral Cortex: The cerebral cortex is the outermost layer of the cerebral hemispheres, characterized by its convoluted surface and distinctive folds called gyri and sulci. It is divided into four lobes: the frontal lobe, parietal lobe, temporal lobe, and occipital lobe. Each lobe is associated with specific functions and contributes to diverse aspects of cognition, perception, and behavior.

Functional Localization: The cerebral cortex exhibits a remarkable degree of functional specialization, with different regions dedicated to specific sensory, motor, and cognitive functions. For example, the primary motor cortex, located in the frontal lobe, controls voluntary movement, while the primary somatosensory cortex, situated in the parietal lobe, processes tactile sensation. Higher-order cognitive functions, such as language and executive function, are mediated by specialized cortical areas distributed across multiple lobes.

White Matter Tracts: Beneath the cerebral cortex lies a network of white matter tracts composed of myelinated axons that facilitate communication between different brain regions. These white matter pathways serve as the neural highways of the brain, transmitting electrical signals and coordinating information processing across distributed neural circuits.

Conclusion: In conclusion, the human brain is a marvel of biological engineering, comprising a complex network of interconnected structures and functional networks that underlie cognition, behavior, and emotion. Understanding the architectural complexity of the brain provides insights into its remarkable capabilities and sheds light on the mechanisms underlying neurological disorders and brain dysfunction. As research continues to unravel the mysteries of brain structure and function, we gain deeper insights into the workings of the mind and the nature of human consciousness.

The Cerebrum: Seat of Higher Cognitive Functions

The cerebrum, the largest and most prominent part of the human brain, is responsible for orchestrating a vast array of cognitive, emotional, and behavioral processes. Comprising the cerebral cortex and underlying white matter, the cerebrum plays a central role in sensory perception, motor control, language, memory, and executive function. In this exploration of the cerebrum, we delve into its structure, organization, and functional significance, unraveling the intricate complexities that underpin human cognition and behavior.

Anatomy of the Cerebrum: The cerebrum is divided into two cerebral hemispheres, each comprising four lobes: the frontal lobe, parietal lobe, temporal lobe, and occipital lobe. These lobes are delineated by prominent sulci and gyri, which increase the surface area of the cerebral cortex and accommodate the vast number of neurons that comprise it. Beneath the cerebral cortex lies a network of white matter tracts that facilitate communication between different regions of the brain.

Functional Localization: Each lobe of the cerebrum is associated with specific functions and contributes to different aspects of cognition and behavior. The frontal lobe, located in the anterior portion of the cerebrum, is involved in executive functions such as decision-making, planning, and impulse control. The parietal lobe, situated posterior to the frontal lobe, is responsible for processing sensory information and spatial awareness. The temporal lobe, located inferior to the frontal and parietal lobes, plays a key role in auditory processing, language comprehension, and memory formation. The occipital lobe, positioned at the back of the cerebrum, is primarily involved in visual processing and perception.

Primary Cortical Areas: Within each lobe of the cerebrum are specialized cortical areas dedicated to specific sensory and motor functions. For example, the primary motor cortex, located in the frontal lobe, controls voluntary movement, with different regions corresponding to specific body parts. The primary somatosensory cortex, situated in the parietal lobe, receives and processes tactile sensation from the body's surface, with a somatotopic organization reflecting the spatial arrangement of sensory receptors. Similarly, the primary auditory cortex in the temporal lobe and the primary visual cortex in the occipital lobe are responsible for processing auditory and visual information, respectively.

Association Cortices: In addition to the primary cortical areas, the cerebrum contains a network of association cortices that integrate sensory inputs, coordinate motor outputs, and support higher-order cognitive functions. These association areas are interconnected with each other and with the primary cortical areas, forming complex neural circuits that underlie perception, memory, attention, language, and problem-solving.

For example, the prefrontal cortex, located in the frontal lobe, is involved in executive functions such as working memory, cognitive flexibility, and social behavior.

Cerebral Hemispheric Lateralization: The two cerebral hemispheres exhibit functional specialization, with each hemisphere contributing unique capabilities to cognitive processing. While both hemispheres are involved in most cognitive functions, certain tasks exhibit hemispheric dominance, with the left hemisphere typically associated with language, logic, and analytical thinking, and the right hemisphere more involved in spatial perception, creativity, and emotional processing. This hemispheric lateralization is evident in patients with split-brain syndrome and provides insights into the organization of cognitive functions in the human brain.

Conclusion: In conclusion, the cerebrum serves as the epicenter of human cognition, housing a diverse array of neural structures and functional networks that underpin sensory perception, motor control, language, memory, and executive function. Understanding the structure and organization of the cerebrum provides insights into the neural basis of human behavior and cognition, shedding light on the complexities of the human mind and brain. As research continues to unravel the mysteries of cerebrum function, we gain deeper insights into the nature of consciousness and the essence of human experience.

The Cerebellum: Master of Coordination and Precision

Nestled beneath the cerebral hemispheres, the cerebellum stands as a vital structure in the brain, playing a crucial role in coordinating movement, maintaining balance, and refining motor skills. Often referred to as the "little brain," the cerebellum comprises intricate neural circuits and specialized cell types that enable precise control and coordination of voluntary movements. In this exploration of the cerebellum, we delve into its anatomy, connectivity, and functional significance, unraveling the remarkable complexities that underlie its role in motor control and cognition.

Anatomy of the Cerebellum: The cerebellum is a compact structure located posterior to the brainstem, dorsal to the fourth ventricle, and inferior to the occipital lobes of the cerebral hemispheres. It consists of two hemispheres, connected by a narrow midline structure called the vermis. The cerebellar cortex, the outermost layer of the cerebellum, is highly convoluted, forming a series of parallel ridges called folia. Beneath the cerebellar cortex lies the cerebellar white matter, which contains myelinated axons that transmit signals between different regions of the cerebellum and other parts of the brain.

Cerebellar Circuitry: The cerebellum contains a complex network of neural circuits organized into distinct anatomical and functional zones. Inputs to the cerebellum originate from the cerebral cortex, brainstem nuclei, and spinal cord, conveying sensory information related to proprioception, balance, and motor commands. These inputs converge onto the cerebellar cortex, where they are processed and integrated by excitatory granule cells and inhibitory Purkinje cells. Output signals from the cerebellum are then transmitted to the motor centers of the brainstem and cerebral cortex, modulating motor commands and refining movement execution.

Functional Significance: The cerebellum plays a central role in motor control and coordination, contributing to the precision, accuracy, and timing of voluntary movements. It is involved in a wide range of motor tasks, including posture control, balance maintenance, gait coordination, and fine motor skills such as handwriting and instrument playing. Dysfunction of the cerebellum can lead to motor impairments and coordination deficits, as observed in conditions such as cerebellar ataxia, dysmetria, and intention tremor.

Cognitive Functions: In addition to its role in motor control, the cerebellum also contributes to cognitive functions such as attention, language, and executive function. Evidence from neuroimaging studies suggests that the cerebellum is involved in non-motor tasks, including working memory, language processing, and emotional regulation. Dysfunction of the cerebellum has been implicated in cognitive deficits observed in cerebellar disorders and neurodevelopmental conditions such as autism spectrum disorder.

Clinical Relevance: Disorders affecting the cerebellum can have profound implications for motor function, cognition, and overall quality of life. Cerebellar lesions, whether due to stroke, trauma, or neurodegenerative diseases, can result in motor deficits such as ataxia, dysmetria, and tremor. Treatment approaches for cerebellar disorders may include physical therapy, pharmacological interventions, and surgical interventions in select cases.

Conclusion: In conclusion, the cerebellum is a remarkable structure in the brain, essential for coordinating movement, maintaining balance, and refining motor skills. Its intricate circuitry and functional connectivity enable precise control and coordination of voluntary movements, contributing to our ability to navigate the world with agility and grace. As our understanding of the cerebellum continues to evolve, so too does our appreciation for its critical role in motor control, cognition, and human behavior.

The Brainstem: Gateway to Vital Functions

The brainstem, often regarded as the "control center" of the central nervous system, serves as a crucial nexus for regulating essential physiological functions and coordinating communication between the brain and the rest of the body. Positioned at the base of the brain, the brainstem integrates sensory inputs, controls autonomic processes, and coordinates motor responses, playing a pivotal role in maintaining homeostasis and ensuring the survival of the organism. In this comprehensive exploration, we delve into the anatomy, functions, and clinical significance of the brainstem, unraveling its remarkable complexity and indispensable role in human physiology.

Anatomy of the Brainstem: The brainstem is a cylindrical structure located between the cerebral hemispheres and the spinal cord, comprising three main regions: the midbrain, pons, and medulla oblongata. Each region exhibits distinct anatomical features and functional properties, contributing to a diverse array of physiological processes.

Midbrain: The midbrain, also known as the mesencephalon, occupies the uppermost portion of the brainstem, connecting the forebrain to the hindbrain. It contains several important structures, including the tectum, tegmentum, and cerebral peduncles. The tectum, comprised of the superior and inferior colliculi, plays a key role in processing visual and auditory information and generating reflexive responses. The tegmentum contains nuclei involved in motor coordination, sensory processing, and arousal.

Pons: Situated between the midbrain and the medulla oblongata, the pons serves as a bridge connecting the cerebellum to the rest of the brain. It contains a complex network of neural pathways involved in motor control, sensory processing, and autonomic regulation. The pons also houses nuclei responsible for controlling facial expressions, eye movements, and respiratory rhythm.

Medulla Oblongata: The medulla oblongata, located at the base of the brainstem, connects the brainstem to the spinal cord and serves as a vital relay center for sensory and motor information. It contains nuclei responsible for regulating autonomic functions such as heart rate, blood pressure, respiration, and digestion. Additionally, the medulla oblongata coordinates reflexive responses, including coughing, sneezing, swallowing, and vomiting.

Functional Significance: The brainstem plays a critical role in regulating essential physiological functions that are necessary for survival and maintaining homeostasis. It serves as the control center for autonomic processes such as heart rate, blood pressure, respiration, and gastrointestinal motility, ensuring the optimal functioning of vital organ systems. Additionally, the brainstem coordinates motor responses, including posture control, balance maintenance, and reflexive movements, enabling adaptive responses to environmental stimuli.

Integration of Sensory Inputs: The brainstem serves as a gateway for processing and integrating sensory inputs from the external environment and the internal milieu. Sensory pathways from the spinal cord, cranial nerves, and higher brain centers converge in the brainstem, where they are processed and relayed to higher cortical regions for further interpretation and response. This integration of sensory information allows for the detection of environmental cues, the initiation of appropriate motor responses, and the maintenance of sensory-motor coordination.

Clinical Relevance: Disorders affecting the brainstem can have profound implications for neurological function and overall health. Lesions or damage to specific brainstem nuclei or pathways can result in a wide range of neurological deficits, including cranial nerve dysfunction, motor impairment, sensory loss, autonomic dysfunction, and alterations in consciousness. Common brainstem disorders include stroke, brainstem tumors, multiple sclerosis, and traumatic brain injury, each presenting unique challenges for diagnosis and management.

Conclusion: In conclusion, the brainstem stands as a vital nexus for regulating essential physiological functions and coordinating communication between the brain and the rest of the body. Its intricate anatomy and functional connectivity enable the integration of sensory inputs, the control of autonomic processes, and the coordination of motor responses, ensuring the survival and well-being of the organism. As our understanding of the brainstem continues to evolve, so too does our appreciation for its indispensable role in human physiology and the complexities of neurological function.

Blood Supply to the Brain: Sustaining the Seat of Consciousness

The brain, the most metabolically active organ in the body, relies on a constant and uninterrupted supply of oxygen and nutrients to support its myriad functions. The intricate network of blood vessels that permeates the brain delivers essential substrates while ensuring the removal of metabolic waste products, playing a pivotal role in maintaining cerebral perfusion and neuronal viability. In this comprehensive exploration, we delve into the anatomy, regulation, and clinical significance of the blood supply to the brain, unraveling the remarkable complexities that sustain the seat of consciousness.

Anatomy of Cerebral Blood Supply: The blood supply to the brain is provided by two pairs of arteries: the internal carotid arteries and the vertebral arteries. The internal carotid arteries, originating from the common carotid arteries, ascend through the neck and enter the skull through the carotid canals, giving rise to the anterior cerebral arteries and the middle cerebral arteries. The vertebral arteries, arising from the subclavian arteries, ascend through the cervical spine and merge to form the basilar artery, which subsequently divides into the posterior cerebral arteries. These arteries supply oxygenated blood to different regions of the brain, ensuring adequate perfusion and metabolic support.

Circle of Willis: The Circle of Willis, a circular anastomosis at the base of the brain, serves as a critical collateral pathway that ensures uninterrupted blood flow to the brain, even in the presence of arterial occlusion or stenosis. It connects the anterior and posterior cerebral circulations via the anterior communicating artery, posterior communicating arteries, and connecting branches between the internal carotid and vertebral arteries. The Circle of Willis provides redundancy and resilience to the cerebral circulation, protecting against ischemic injury and maintaining cerebral perfusion pressure.

Regulation of Cerebral Blood Flow: Cerebral blood flow is tightly regulated by a complex interplay of neural, metabolic, and vascular mechanisms that maintain adequate perfusion to meet the metabolic demands of the brain. Autoregulation, the ability of cerebral blood vessels to adjust their diameter in response to changes in cerebral perfusion pressure, ensures a constant blood flow over a wide range of systemic blood pressures. Neurovascular coupling, the coupling of neuronal activity to local changes in blood flow, ensures that regions of increased neuronal activity receive enhanced perfusion to meet their metabolic demands. Additionally, neurohumoral factors such as carbon dioxide, oxygen, and pH levels modulate cerebral blood flow by affecting vascular tone and diameter.

Clinical Implications: Disorders affecting the blood supply to the brain can have profound implications for neurological function and overall health. Ischemic stroke, resulting from arterial occlusion or stenosis, deprives brain tissue of oxygen and nutrients, leading to neuronal injury and neurological deficits. Hemorrhagic stroke, caused by rupture of blood vessels within the brain, results in intracerebral bleeding and increased intracranial pressure, posing a life-threatening emergency. Other conditions affecting cerebral blood flow include transient ischemic attacks, cerebral aneurysms, arteriovenous malformations, and vasospasm following subarachnoid hemorrhage.

Therapeutic Interventions: Therapeutic interventions aimed at restoring or maintaining cerebral perfusion play a crucial role in the management of cerebrovascular disorders. Acute ischemic stroke may be treated with thrombolytic therapy or mechanical thrombectomy to restore blood flow and salvage ischemic brain tissue. Hemorrhagic stroke requires prompt management to control bleeding and reduce intracranial pressure, often involving surgical interventions such as craniotomy or endovascular coiling. Additionally, preventive measures such as anticoagulation, antiplatelet therapy, blood pressure control, and lifestyle modifications can reduce the risk of stroke and optimize cerebral perfusion.

Conclusion: In conclusion, the blood supply to the brain is a complex and intricately regulated system that sustains the metabolic demands of the most vital organ in the body. The intricate network of arteries, arterioles, capillaries, and veins ensures the delivery of oxygen and nutrients to every corner of the brain while maintaining homeostasis and removing metabolic waste products. Understanding the anatomy, regulation, and clinical significance of cerebral blood flow is essential for diagnosing and managing cerebrovascular disorders and optimizing neurological outcomes. As research continues to unravel the mysteries of cerebral perfusion, new insights into the pathophysiology of cerebrovascular disease and innovative therapeutic approaches promise to revolutionize the care of patients with neurological disorders.

The Blood-Brain Barrier: Guardian of Neural Integrity

The blood-brain barrier (BBB) stands as a formidable barrier that safeguards the delicate neural tissue of the brain from the external milieu, regulating the passage of substances between the bloodstream and the central nervous system. Comprising specialized endothelial cells, tight junctions, and astrocytic foot processes, the BBB plays a pivotal role in maintaining cerebral homeostasis, protecting against neurotoxic substances, and facilitating the transport of essential nutrients to support neuronal function. In this comprehensive exploration, we delve into the anatomy, physiology, regulation, and clinical significance of the blood-brain barrier, unraveling the remarkable complexities that underlie its role as the guardian of neural integrity.

Anatomy of the Blood-Brain Barrier: The blood-brain barrier is formed by a complex interplay of cellular and molecular components that restrict the passage of substances between the blood and the brain parenchyma. The primary cellular component of the BBB is the specialized endothelial cells that line the capillaries within the brain. These endothelial cells are interconnected by tight junctions, which create a physical barrier that prevents the diffusion of hydrophilic molecules and large molecules from crossing the endothelial layer. Additionally, astrocytic end-feet ensheath the cerebral blood vessels, providing structural support and releasing signaling molecules that regulate BBB integrity and function.

Functions of the Blood-Brain Barrier: The blood-brain barrier serves multiple crucial functions that are essential for maintaining cerebral homeostasis and preserving neural integrity. It regulates the passage of ions, nutrients, and metabolic substrates into the brain, ensuring the provision of essential molecules necessary for neuronal function and energy metabolism. Conversely, it restricts the entry of potentially harmful substances, including toxins, pathogens, and neuroactive compounds, thereby protecting the brain from neurotoxicity and infection. Additionally, the BBB plays a role in maintaining the composition of the cerebral microenvironment, regulating ion concentrations, pH levels, and osmotic balance within the brain parenchyma.

Regulation of Blood-Brain Barrier Function: The integrity and permeability of the blood-brain barrier are regulated by a complex interplay of cellular, molecular, and physiological mechanisms. Endothelial cells express a variety of transporters, receptors, and efflux pumps that actively regulate the transport of substances across the BBB. Astrocytes release signaling molecules, such as glial-derived neurotrophic factor (GDNF) and transforming growth factor-beta (TGF-β), which modulate tight junction protein expression and maintain BBB integrity. Additionally, neuroinflammatory mediators, such as cytokines and chemokines, can disrupt BBB function and increase permeability, contributing to neuroinflammation and neurodegenerative diseases.

Clinical Implications: Disruption of blood-brain barrier function has been implicated in the pathogenesis of various neurological disorders, including neurodegenerative diseases, inflammatory conditions, and brain tumors. In neurodegenerative diseases such as Alzheimer's disease and Parkinson's disease, BBB dysfunction allows the infiltration of neurotoxic proteins, inflammatory mediators, and immune cells into the brain, exacerbating neuronal injury and disease progression. Similarly, in inflammatory conditions such as multiple sclerosis and autoimmune encephalitis, breakdown of the BBB leads to immune cell infiltration, demyelination, and neuroinflammation. Additionally, disruption of the BBB in brain tumors facilitates tumor growth, invasion, and metastasis, posing challenges for targeted drug delivery and therapeutic intervention.

Therapeutic Strategies: Therapeutic strategies aimed at modulating blood-brain barrier function hold promise for the treatment of neurological disorders and improving drug delivery to the brain. Drug delivery systems, such as nanoparticles, liposomes, and cell-penetrating peptides, can bypass the BBB and deliver therapeutics directly to the brain parenchyma, enhancing drug efficacy and reducing systemic side effects. Additionally, targeted approaches to modulate BBB permeability, such as focused ultrasound, osmotic disruption, and pharmacological agents, offer potential avenues for enhancing drug delivery and improving therapeutic outcomes in neurological diseases.

Conclusion: In conclusion, the blood-brain barrier is a remarkable physiological barrier that protects the brain from the external environment, maintains cerebral homeostasis, and preserves neural integrity. Its intricate anatomy, regulation, and function ensure the selective transport of essential nutrients while preventing the entry of harmful substances into the brain parenchyma. Understanding the complexities of the blood-brain barrier is essential for elucidating the pathophysiology of neurological disorders and developing innovative therapeutic strategies aimed at preserving neural function and improving patient outcomes. As research continues to unravel the mysteries of BBB biology, new insights into its role in health and disease promise to revolutionize the field of neurology and advance our understanding of the human brain.

Neuroglia: Unsung Heroes of Brain Function and Health

While neurons have long been regarded as the stars of the central nervous system, a closer look reveals a diverse cast of supporting characters that play equally vital roles in brain function and health. Enter neuroglia, the unsung heroes of the brain, comprising a multitude of specialized cells that provide structural support, regulate neuronal activity, and maintain homeostasis within the central nervous system. In this comprehensive exploration, we delve into the anatomy, functions, and clinical significance of neuroglia, shedding light on their indispensable contributions to brain function and overall neurological well-being.

Anatomy of Neuroglia: Neuroglia, also known as glial cells or simply glia, are non-neuronal cells that outnumber neurons in the central nervous system by a ratio of approximately 10 to 1. They are classified into several distinct types, each with unique morphological and functional characteristics. The main types of neuroglia include astrocytes, oligodendrocytes, microglia, and ependymal cells.

Astrocytes: Astrocytes are star-shaped glial cells that form intimate associations with neurons and blood vessels, playing diverse roles in neuronal signaling, synaptic transmission, and metabolic support. They regulate extracellular ion concentrations, recycle neurotransmitters, and provide neurons with energy substrates such as glucose and lactate. Additionally, astrocytes play a critical role in maintaining the blood-brain barrier, modulating synaptic plasticity, and responding to injury and inflammation in the central nervous system.

Oligodendrocytes: Oligodendrocytes are glial cells responsible for producing myelin, a lipid-rich insulating sheath that wraps around neuronal axons to facilitate rapid conduction of electrical impulses. Myelination increases the efficiency and speed of neuronal communication, allowing for faster transmission of signals across long distances within the central nervous system. Dysfunction of oligodendrocytes or demyelination can impair neuronal signaling and lead to neurological disorders such as multiple sclerosis.

Microglia: Microglia are the resident immune cells of the central nervous system, surveilling the brain parenchyma for signs of injury, infection, or inflammation. Upon activation, microglia undergo morphological changes and release inflammatory mediators, phagocytosing cellular debris, pathogens, and abnormal proteins. While microglia play a crucial role in host defense and tissue repair, dysregulated microglial activation has been implicated in neuroinflammatory diseases and neurodegenerative disorders.

Ependymal Cells: Ependymal cells line the ventricles of the brain and the central canal of the spinal cord, forming a barrier between the cerebrospinal fluid and the brain parenchyma. They produce cerebrospinal fluid, which serves as a cushioning and protective fluid that surrounds the brain and spinal cord. Additionally, ependymal cells contribute to the regulation of cerebrospinal fluid dynamics and the maintenance of brain volume and intracranial pressure.

Functions of Neuroglia: Neuroglia play diverse and essential roles in supporting neuronal function, maintaining homeostasis, and preserving overall brain health. They provide structural support and insulation for neurons, regulate extracellular ion concentrations, and modulate synaptic transmission and plasticity. Additionally, neuroglia participate in the maintenance of the blood-brain barrier, the clearance of metabolic waste products, and the regulation of neuroinflammatory responses. Moreover, recent evidence suggests that neuroglia may also play roles in neurogenesis, synaptic pruning, and the modulation of neural circuits during development and adulthood.

Clinical Significance: Dysfunction or dysregulation of neuroglial cells has been implicated in a wide range of neurological disorders and neurodegenerative diseases. Astrocyte dysfunction has been associated with epilepsy, Alzheimer's disease, and amyotrophic lateral sclerosis (ALS), while oligodendrocyte dysfunction and demyelination are hallmark features of multiple sclerosis. Microglial activation and neuroinflammation have been implicated in Parkinson's disease, Huntington's disease, and Alzheimer's disease, contributing to neurodegeneration and disease progression. Additionally, disruptions in ependymal cell function have been linked to hydrocephalus, a condition characterized by the accumulation of cerebrospinal fluid within the brain ventricles.

Conclusion: In conclusion, neuroglia are indispensable players in brain function and health, supporting neuronal function, maintaining homeostasis, and preserving overall neurological well-being. Their diverse roles in structural support, metabolic regulation, synaptic transmission, and immune defense underscore their importance in orchestrating the complex activities of the central nervous system. As our understanding of neuroglia continues to evolve, so too does our appreciation for their essential contributions to brain function and the pathophysiology of neurological disorders. Further research into the biology of neuroglia promises to yield insights into the mechanisms of neurological disease and novel therapeutic strategies for preserving neural function and combating neurological disorders.

Glioblastoma and Neuroanatomy: Insights into Tumor Localization and Impact

Glioblastoma, the most aggressive and malignant form of glioma, presents a formidable challenge to both patients and clinicians due to its infiltrative nature and resistance to conventional therapies. Understanding the intricate relationship between glioblastoma and neuroanatomy is crucial for elucidating tumor localization, characterizing clinical manifestations, and devising targeted treatment strategies. In this comprehensive exploration, we delve into the neuroanatomical correlates of glioblastoma, unraveling the complex interplay between tumor biology and brain structure, and highlighting the implications for diagnosis, prognosis, and therapeutic intervention.

Anatomy of the Brain: The brain, the most complex organ in the human body, comprises distinct regions and structures that govern a myriad of physiological functions and cognitive processes. Major anatomical divisions include the cerebrum, cerebellum, and brainstem, each contributing to sensory perception, motor control, and higher-order cognitive functions. The cerebral cortex, with its convoluted surface and intricate neural networks, is particularly susceptible to the development of glioblastoma, given its high metabolic activity and dense cellular composition.

Localization of Glioblastoma: Glioblastoma typically arises within the cerebral hemispheres, particularly in regions of the brain with abundant glial cell populations, such as the frontal, temporal, and parietal lobes. Tumor localization may vary depending on genetic mutations, cellular origin, and microenvironmental factors, with preferential involvement of specific brain regions influencing clinical presentation and treatment outcomes. Glioblastoma exhibits infiltrative growth patterns, diffusely infiltrating adjacent brain tissue and crossing anatomical boundaries, making complete surgical resection challenging and contributing to high rates of tumor recurrence.

Impact on Neuroanatomy: Glioblastoma exerts profound effects on neuroanatomy, disrupting normal brain structure and function through mass effect, compression of adjacent structures, and infiltration of tumor cells into surrounding parenchyma. Tumor growth can lead to increased intracranial pressure, displacement of normal brain tissue, and distortion of anatomical landmarks, resulting in neurological deficits such as seizures, focal motor weakness, sensory disturbances, and cognitive impairment. Additionally, peritumoral edema and vasogenic changes further exacerbate neuroanatomical alterations, contributing to clinical morbidity and disease progression.

Neuroimaging Correlates: Neuroimaging modalities such as magnetic resonance imaging (MRI) play a crucial role in localizing glioblastoma lesions, characterizing tumor morphology, and assessing treatment response. Contrast-enhanced MRI reveals ring-enhancing lesions with central necrosis, reflecting the highly proliferative nature of glioblastoma and the disruption of the blood-brain barrier. Diffusion-weighted imaging (DWI) and perfusion-weighted imaging (PWI) provide insights into tumor cellularity, vascularity, and microstructural changes, aiding in treatment planning and prognostication.

Clinical Considerations: Understanding the neuroanatomical correlates of glioblastoma is essential for guiding clinical management decisions and optimizing patient outcomes. Surgical resection, often combined with adjuvant radiation and chemotherapy, aims to achieve maximal tumor debulking while preserving critical neuroanatomical structures and minimizing postoperative deficits. Advanced neuroimaging techniques, such as functional MRI (fMRI) and intraoperative neuronavigation, assist in surgical planning and intraoperative mapping of eloquent brain regions, reducing the risk of neurological complications and maximizing extent of resection.

Future Directions: Advances in molecular profiling, imaging technology, and targeted therapies hold promise for improving the diagnosis and treatment of glioblastoma by incorporating neuroanatomical considerations into personalized treatment algorithms. Integration of genomic biomarkers, such as IDH mutation status and MGMT promoter methylation, with neuroanatomical imaging data may enable more accurate prognostication and treatment stratification. Additionally, innovative approaches such as immunotherapy, targeted drug delivery, and gene editing techniques offer potential avenues for enhancing therapeutic efficacy and prolonging survival in patients with glioblastoma.

Conclusion: In conclusion, the intricate interplay between glioblastoma and neuroanatomy underscores the complexity of tumor localization, clinical manifestation, and therapeutic response. By elucidating the neuroanatomical correlates of glioblastoma, clinicians can better understand the impact of tumor growth on brain structure and function, tailor treatment strategies to individual patients, and improve outcomes for this devastating disease. Further research into the molecular mechanisms and neurobiological underpinnings of glioblastoma promises to unlock new insights into disease pathogenesis and therapeutic targets, offering hope for the development of more effective treatments and ultimately, a cure for this aggressive brain tumor.

CHAPTER 3: PATHOGENESIS OF GLIOBLASTOMA

Genetic Alterations and Molecular Pathways in Glioblastoma: Unraveling the Molecular Complexity

Glioblastoma, the most aggressive and lethal form of primary brain tumor, is characterized by a complex interplay of genetic alterations and dysregulated molecular pathways that drive tumorigenesis, invasion, and therapeutic resistance. Understanding the molecular landscape of glioblastoma is essential for elucidating disease pathogenesis, identifying prognostic markers, and developing targeted therapies aimed at improving patient outcomes. In this comprehensive exploration, we delve into the genetic alterations and molecular pathways implicated in glioblastoma, unraveling the intricate mechanisms underlying tumor initiation, progression, and therapeutic resistance.

Genetic Alterations in Glioblastoma: Glioblastoma is characterized by extensive genetic heterogeneity, with recurrent alterations affecting key oncogenes, tumor suppressor genes, and signaling pathways. Prominent genetic alterations observed in glioblastoma include mutations in the tumor suppressor genes TP53, PTEN, and RB1, which disrupt cell cycle regulation, apoptosis, and DNA repair mechanisms, leading to uncontrolled cell proliferation and genomic instability. Additionally, amplifications and overexpression of oncogenes such as EGFR, PDGFRA, and PIK3CA drive aberrant signaling cascades that promote cell survival, proliferation, and invasion.

Molecular Pathways Implicated in Glioblastoma: Glioblastoma is characterized by dysregulated molecular pathways that govern cell growth, survival, invasion, and angiogenesis. The receptor tyrosine kinase (RTK)/RAS/PI3K pathway is frequently dysregulated in glioblastoma, with mutations and amplifications affecting RTKs such as EGFR and PDGFRA, leading to constitutive activation of downstream signaling cascades involved in cell proliferation and survival. The phosphatidylinositol 3-kinase (PI3K)/AKT/mTOR pathway plays a central role in promoting cell growth and inhibiting apoptosis, with dysregulation contributing to glioblastoma progression and therapeutic resistance.

Epigenetic Alterations: In addition to genetic mutations, glioblastoma exhibits widespread epigenetic alterations that contribute to tumor initiation, progression, and therapy resistance. DNA methylation, histone modifications, and chromatin remodeling play crucial roles in regulating gene expression patterns and cellular phenotypes in glioblastoma. Aberrant DNA methylation patterns, in particular, have been implicated in silencing tumor suppressor genes and promoting oncogenic signaling pathways, contributing to gliomagenesis and treatment resistance.

Tumor Microenvironment: The tumor microenvironment plays a critical role in glioblastoma pathobiology, influencing tumor growth, invasion, and therapeutic response. Glioblastoma-associated microglia and macrophages (GAMs) are recruited to the tumor site, where they contribute to tumor progression through secretion of cytokines, growth factors, and extracellular matrix remodeling enzymes. Additionally, interactions between glioma cells and components of the tumor microenvironment, such as endothelial cells, pericytes, and astrocytes, promote tumor angiogenesis, immune evasion, and therapeutic resistance.

Therapeutic Implications: Understanding the genetic alterations and molecular pathways driving glioblastoma is essential for developing targeted therapeutic strategies aimed at disrupting oncogenic signaling cascades and overcoming treatment resistance. Targeted therapies directed against specific molecular targets, such as EGFR inhibitors, PI3K inhibitors, and angiogenesis inhibitors, have shown promise in preclinical studies and early-phase clinical trials. Additionally, immunotherapy approaches, including immune checkpoint inhibitors and chimeric antigen receptor (CAR) T cell therapy, hold potential for harnessing the immune system to target glioblastoma cells and improve patient outcomes.

Challenges and Future Directions: Despite significant advances in our understanding of the molecular landscape of glioblastoma, challenges remain in translating this knowledge into effective therapeutic interventions that improve patient outcomes. Tumor heterogeneity, therapeutic resistance, and the complex interplay between genetic and environmental factors pose formidable obstacles to successful treatment. Future research efforts aimed at elucidating the dynamic interplay between genetic alterations, molecular pathways, and the tumor microenvironment will be essential for identifying novel therapeutic targets and developing personalized treatment strategies for patients with glioblastoma.

Conclusion: In conclusion, glioblastoma is characterized by extensive genetic alterations and dysregulated molecular pathways that drive tumor initiation, progression, and therapeutic resistance. Understanding the molecular complexity of glioblastoma is essential for identifying novel therapeutic targets and developing personalized treatment strategies aimed at improving patient outcomes. Further research efforts focused on unraveling the intricate mechanisms underlying glioblastoma pathogenesis and treatment resistance hold promise for revolutionizing the management of this devastating disease and ultimately, improving patient survival and quality of life.

The Tumor Microenvironment in Glioblastoma: A Dynamic Landscape of Interactions

Glioblastoma, characterized by its aggressive growth and infiltrative nature, thrives within a complex and dynamic microenvironment that encompasses a multitude of cellular and molecular components. The tumor microenvironment (TME) plays a pivotal role in glioblastoma pathogenesis, driving tumor growth, invasion, angiogenesis, and therapeutic resistance. Understanding the intricate interactions within the TME is essential for elucidating disease progression mechanisms, identifying therapeutic targets, and developing novel treatment strategies. In this comprehensive exploration, we delve into the cellular and molecular constituents of the glioblastoma TME, unraveling its complexity and highlighting its significance in disease biology and clinical management.

Cellular Components of the Tumor Microenvironment: The TME of glioblastoma is comprised of a diverse array of cell types, including tumor cells, immune cells, stromal cells, and vascular cells, each contributing to tumor growth and progression through intricate interactions and crosstalk. Glioma cells, the primary constituents of the tumor mass, exhibit heterogeneity in genetic and phenotypic characteristics, driving tumor initiation, invasion, and therapeutic resistance. Immune cells such as microglia, macrophages, T cells, and regulatory T cells (Tregs) infiltrate the glioblastoma microenvironment, exerting both pro-tumorigenic and anti-tumorigenic effects depending on their activation status and functional phenotype. Additionally, stromal cells such as cancer-associated fibroblasts (CAFs) and endothelial cells contribute to tumor progression by promoting angiogenesis, extracellular matrix remodeling, and immunosuppression.

Molecular Signaling Pathways in the Tumor

Microenvironment: The TME of glioblastoma is characterized by dysregulated molecular signaling pathways that promote tumor growth, invasion, and therapeutic resistance. The receptor tyrosine kinase (RTK)/RAS/PI3K pathway plays a central role in glioblastoma pathogenesis, with aberrant activation of RTKs such as EGFR and PDGFRA driving downstream signaling cascades involved in cell proliferation, survival, and migration. Additionally, the phosphatidylinositol 3-kinase (PI3K)/AKT/mTOR pathway regulates key cellular processes such as metabolism, apoptosis, and autophagy, contributing to glioblastoma growth and therapeutic resistance. Dysregulated immune signaling pathways, such as the PD-1/PD-L1 axis and the TGF-β signaling pathway, promote immunosuppression within the TME, enabling tumor immune evasion and progression.

Extracellular Matrix and Tumor-Stroma Interactions: The extracellular matrix (ECM) serves as a scaffold for tumor growth and invasion within the TME, providing physical support and modulating cellular behavior through biochemical signaling cues. Remodeling of the ECM by glioblastoma cells and stromal cells promotes tumor invasion, angiogenesis, and metastasis, facilitating the spread of tumor cells into surrounding brain tissue and distant sites. Interactions between glioblastoma cells and stromal cells within the TME, mediated by cell adhesion molecules, growth factors, and cytokines, further contribute to tumor progression and therapeutic resistance.

Angiogenesis and Vascular Remodeling: Angiogenesis, the process of new blood vessel formation, plays a critical role in glioblastoma growth and progression by supplying oxygen and nutrients to the expanding tumor mass. Dysregulated angiogenic signaling pathways, such as the vascular endothelial growth factor (VEGF) pathway, promote aberrant vessel formation and vascular permeability within the TME, leading to tumor hypoxia, necrosis, and therapeutic resistance. Additionally, vascular remodeling and co-option of pre-existing blood vessels by glioblastoma cells contribute to tumor invasion and dissemination, further complicating therapeutic intervention.

Therapeutic Implications: Targeting the TME represents a promising strategy for improving the efficacy of glioblastoma therapy and overcoming treatment resistance. Therapeutic approaches aimed at disrupting tumor-stroma interactions, modulating immune signaling pathways, and inhibiting angiogenesis have shown promise in preclinical studies and early-phase clinical trials. Immunotherapy strategies, including immune checkpoint inhibitors, chimeric antigen receptor (CAR) T cell therapy, and dendritic cell vaccines, aim to harness the host immune system to target glioblastoma cells and enhance anti-tumor immune responses within the TME. Additionally, anti-angiogenic agents targeting VEGF and other pro-angiogenic factors have demonstrated efficacy in inhibiting tumor growth and improving patient survival.

Challenges and Future Directions: Despite significant advances in our understanding of the TME in glioblastoma, challenges remain in translating this knowledge into effective therapeutic interventions that improve patient outcomes. Tumor heterogeneity, therapeutic resistance, and the dynamic nature of the TME pose formidable obstacles to successful treatment. Future research efforts aimed at elucidating the molecular mechanisms underlying TME interactions, identifying novel therapeutic targets, and developing combination treatment strategies hold promise for revolutionizing the management of glioblastoma and improving patient survival and quality of life.

Conclusion: In conclusion, the tumor microenvironment of glioblastoma represents a complex and dynamic ecosystem of cellular and molecular interactions that drive tumor growth, invasion, and therapeutic resistance. Understanding the intricacies of the TME is essential for elucidating disease pathogenesis, identifying therapeutic targets, and developing novel treatment strategies aimed at improving patient outcomes. Further research into the molecular mechanisms and cellular dynamics within the TME holds promise for advancing our understanding of glioblastoma biology and revolutionizing the management of this devastating disease.

The Role of Inflammation in Glioblastoma: Unraveling the Complex Interplay

Inflammation, traditionally recognized as a protective response to tissue injury and infection, emerges as a critical player in the pathobiology of glioblastoma, the most aggressive primary brain tumor. While inflammation is a fundamental component of the immune response aimed at eliminating pathogens and promoting tissue repair, dysregulated and chronic inflammation within the tumor microenvironment contributes to glioblastoma initiation, progression, and therapeutic resistance. In this comprehensive exploration, we delve into the multifaceted role of inflammation in glioblastoma, elucidating its diverse mechanisms, clinical implications, and therapeutic opportunities.

Inflammatory Mediators in Glioblastoma: The glioblastoma microenvironment is characterized by a milieu of inflammatory mediators, including cytokines, chemokines, growth factors, and reactive oxygen species, which orchestrate a complex network of cellular interactions and signaling pathways. Pro-inflammatory cytokines such as interleukin-6 (IL-6), tumor necrosis factor-alpha (TNF-α), and interleukin-1 beta (IL-1β) promote tumor growth, invasion, and angiogenesis by activating pro-tumorigenic signaling pathways and recruiting immune cells to the tumor site. Additionally, chemokines such as CCL2 and CXCL12 play crucial roles in immune cell recruitment, tumor cell migration, and metastasis, contributing to glioblastoma aggressiveness and treatment resistance.

Immune Cell Infiltration: Immune cells infiltrate the glioblastoma microenvironment, exerting both pro-tumorigenic and anti-tumorigenic effects depending on their functional phenotype and activation status. Microglia and macrophages, the resident immune cells of the central nervous system, play a central role in glioblastoma pathogenesis by promoting tumor growth, invasion, and immunosuppression. Tumor-associated macrophages (TAMs) polarize towards an immunosuppressive M2-like phenotype, secreting anti-inflammatory cytokines and growth factors that promote tumor progression and therapeutic resistance. Additionally, T cells, natural killer (NK) cells, and dendritic cells infiltrate the glioblastoma microenvironment, engaging in dynamic interactions with tumor cells and modulating anti-tumor immune responses.

NF-κB Signaling Pathway: The nuclear factor-kappa B (NF-κB) signaling pathway emerges as a central regulator of inflammation in glioblastoma, orchestrating a diverse array of cellular responses to inflammatory stimuli. NF-κB activation promotes glioblastoma cell survival, proliferation, and invasion by inducing the expression of pro-inflammatory cytokines, anti-apoptotic factors, and angiogenic factors. Dysregulated NF-κB signaling contributes to tumor immune evasion, therapy resistance, and poor clinical outcomes in glioblastoma patients, highlighting its significance as a potential therapeutic target.

Clinical Implications: Inflammation exerts profound effects on glioblastoma biology and clinical outcomes, influencing tumor aggressiveness, therapeutic response, and patient survival. Elevated levels of inflammatory mediators within the glioblastoma microenvironment correlate with poor prognosis and reduced overall survival in patients, underscoring the clinical significance of inflammation as a prognostic biomarker. Additionally, inflammation contributes to treatment resistance by promoting tumor immune evasion, supporting tumor cell survival, and enhancing the stemness and invasiveness of glioblastoma cells. Targeting inflammation represents a promising therapeutic strategy for improving patient outcomes and overcoming treatment resistance in glioblastoma.

Therapeutic Opportunities: Therapeutic interventions aimed at modulating inflammation hold promise for improving the efficacy of current treatment modalities and enhancing patient survival in glioblastoma. Immunotherapy approaches, including immune checkpoint inhibitors, chimeric antigen receptor (CAR) T cell therapy, and dendritic cell vaccines, aim to harness the host immune system to target glioblastoma cells and enhance anti-tumor immune responses within the tumor microenvironment. Additionally, targeting pro-inflammatory signaling pathways such as NF-κB and cytokine signaling pathways may offer opportunities for disrupting tumor-promoting inflammation and sensitizing glioblastoma cells to conventional therapies.

Future Directions: Despite significant advances in our understanding of the role of inflammation in glioblastoma, challenges remain in translating this knowledge into effective therapeutic interventions that improve patient outcomes. Tumor heterogeneity, immune cell plasticity, and the dynamic nature of the glioblastoma microenvironment pose formidable obstacles to successful treatment. Future research efforts aimed at elucidating the molecular mechanisms underlying inflammation in glioblastoma, identifying novel therapeutic targets, and developing combination treatment strategies hold promise for revolutionizing the management of this devastating disease and improving patient survival and quality of life.

Conclusion: In conclusion, inflammation emerges as a critical determinant of glioblastoma pathogenesis, influencing tumor growth, invasion, therapeutic response, and patient outcomes. Understanding the complex interplay between inflammation and glioblastoma biology is essential for developing targeted therapeutic strategies aimed at modulating inflammation and improving patient outcomes. Further research into the molecular mechanisms underlying inflammation in glioblastoma holds promise for identifying novel therapeutic targets and developing innovative treatment approaches that harness the host immune system to combat this devastating disease.

Angiogenesis in Glioblastoma: The Lifeline of Tumor Growth and Progression

Glioblastoma, the most aggressive and lethal form of primary brain tumor, relies on angiogenesis, the process of new blood vessel formation, to sustain its rapid growth, invasion, and progression. Angiogenesis in glioblastoma is a complex and tightly regulated process orchestrated by a myriad of molecular signals and cellular interactions within the tumor microenvironment. Understanding the mechanisms of angiogenesis in glioblastoma is essential for elucidating disease pathogenesis, identifying therapeutic targets, and developing novel treatment strategies aimed at disrupting tumor vasculature and improving patient outcomes. In this comprehensive exploration, we delve into the multifaceted role of angiogenesis in glioblastoma, unraveling its molecular mechanisms, clinical implications, and therapeutic opportunities.

Molecular Mechanisms of Angiogenesis: Angiogenesis in glioblastoma is driven by a complex interplay of pro-angiogenic and anti-angiogenic factors that regulate endothelial cell proliferation, migration, and tube formation. Vascular endothelial growth factor (VEGF), a potent pro-angiogenic cytokine, plays a central role in glioblastoma angiogenesis by promoting endothelial cell survival, proliferation, and vascular permeability. Dysregulated expression of VEGF and its receptors, particularly VEGFR2, leads to aberrant vessel formation and leaky, disorganized vasculature within the tumor microenvironment. Additionally, other pro-angiogenic factors such as basic fibroblast growth factor (bFGF), angiopoietins, and matrix metalloproteinases (MMPs) contribute to glioblastoma angiogenesis through diverse signaling pathways.

Hypoxia and HIF-1α Signaling: Hypoxia, a hallmark feature of solid tumors including glioblastoma, serves as a potent stimulus for angiogenesis by inducing the expression of hypoxia-inducible factor 1-alpha (HIF-1α), a key transcription factor that regulates the expression of genes involved in angiogenesis and oxygen homeostasis. Under hypoxic conditions, HIF-1α promotes the transcription of VEGF and other pro-angiogenic factors, facilitating the formation of new blood vessels to restore oxygen and nutrient supply to the tumor microenvironment. Dysregulated HIF-1α signaling contributes to glioblastoma aggressiveness, therapeutic resistance, and poor clinical outcomes, highlighting its significance as a potential therapeutic target.

Tumor Endothelial Cells and Pericytes: The endothelial cells lining tumor blood vessels in glioblastoma exhibit distinct phenotypic and functional characteristics compared to normal endothelial cells, contributing to tumor angiogenesis and therapeutic resistance. Tumor endothelial cells undergo phenotypic changes, including increased proliferation, migration, and resistance to apoptosis, in response to pro-angiogenic signals within the tumor microenvironment. Additionally, pericytes, specialized mural cells that surround and support endothelial cells, play a crucial role in stabilizing blood vessels and regulating angiogenesis in glioblastoma. Dysregulated interactions between tumor endothelial cells and pericytes contribute to abnormal vessel formation, leaky vasculature, and tumor progression.

Clinical Implications of Angiogenesis: Angiogenesis plays a central role in glioblastoma biology and clinical outcomes, influencing tumor aggressiveness, therapeutic response, and patient survival. Elevated levels of angiogenic factors such as VEGF within the glioblastoma microenvironment correlate with poor prognosis and reduced overall survival in patients, underscoring the clinical significance of angiogenesis as a prognostic biomarker. Additionally, angiogenesis contributes to therapeutic resistance by promoting tumor vascularization, hypoxia-induced radioresistance, and reduced drug delivery to the tumor site. Targeting angiogenesis represents a promising therapeutic strategy for improving patient outcomes and overcoming treatment resistance in glioblastoma.

Therapeutic Opportunities: Therapeutic interventions aimed at targeting angiogenesis hold promise for improving the efficacy of current treatment modalities and enhancing patient survival in glioblastoma. Anti-angiogenic agents targeting VEGF and its receptors, such as bevacizumab and aflibercept, have demonstrated efficacy in inhibiting tumor angiogenesis, reducing tumor vascularization, and improving progression-free survival in glioblastoma patients. Additionally, combination therapies targeting multiple angiogenic pathways, such as VEGF and PDGF signaling, may offer synergistic effects and overcome treatment resistance in glioblastoma.

Future Directions: Despite significant advances in anti-angiogenic therapy for glioblastoma, challenges remain in translating this knowledge into effective therapeutic interventions that improve patient outcomes. Tumor heterogeneity, acquired resistance to anti-angiogenic agents, and the dynamic nature of the tumor microenvironment pose formidable obstacles to successful treatment. Future research efforts aimed at elucidating the molecular mechanisms underlying angiogenesis in glioblastoma, identifying novel therapeutic targets, and developing combination treatment strategies hold promise for revolutionizing the management of this devastating disease and improving patient survival and quality of life.

Conclusion: In conclusion, angiogenesis emerges as a critical determinant of glioblastoma growth, invasion, and progression, influencing tumor aggressiveness, therapeutic response, and patient outcomes. Understanding the molecular mechanisms of angiogenesis in glioblastoma is essential for developing targeted therapeutic strategies aimed at disrupting tumor vasculature and improving patient outcomes. Further research into the complexities of angiogenesis in glioblastoma holds promise for identifying novel therapeutic targets and developing innovative treatment approaches that target the lifeline of tumor growth and progression.

Metabolic Reprogramming in Glioblastoma: Fueling Tumor Growth and Therapeutic Resistance

Glioblastoma, characterized by its relentless growth and resistance to treatment, undergoes metabolic reprogramming to sustain its energy demands, biosynthetic requirements, and survival under adverse conditions. Metabolic alterations in glioblastoma cells enable them to adapt to the unique microenvironment of the central nervous system, evade immune surveillance, and thrive in the face of therapeutic challenges. Understanding the intricacies of metabolic reprogramming in glioblastoma is essential for elucidating disease pathogenesis, identifying therapeutic vulnerabilities, and developing novel treatment strategies aimed at targeting metabolic dependencies. In this comprehensive exploration, we delve into the multifaceted role of metabolic reprogramming in glioblastoma, unraveling its molecular mechanisms, clinical implications, and therapeutic opportunities.

Warburg Effect and Aerobic Glycolysis: Glioblastoma cells exhibit enhanced glycolytic metabolism, a phenomenon known as the Warburg effect, characterized by increased glucose uptake and fermentation of glucose to lactate even in the presence of oxygen. Aerobic glycolysis provides rapid ATP production and metabolic intermediates for biosynthetic pathways, supporting the proliferative and invasive phenotype of glioblastoma cells. Dysregulated expression of glycolytic enzymes, glucose transporters, and oncogenic signaling pathways, such as PI3K/AKT and MYC, contributes to aerobic glycolysis in glioblastoma, promoting tumor growth and therapeutic resistance.

Glutamine Metabolism: In addition to glucose metabolism, glioblastoma cells rely on glutamine as a major carbon and nitrogen source to sustain proliferation and survival. Glutamine is metabolized through the tricarboxylic acid (TCA) cycle to generate ATP, reduce equivalents, and biosynthetic precursors for nucleotide and lipid synthesis. Dysregulated expression of glutamine transporters, glutaminase enzymes, and oncogenic signaling pathways, such as c-Myc and mTOR, enhances glutamine dependency in glioblastoma cells, promoting tumor growth and therapeutic resistance.

Lipid Metabolism: Glioblastoma cells exhibit altered lipid metabolism, characterized by increased lipogenesis, lipid uptake, and fatty acid oxidation to meet the demands of rapid cell proliferation and membrane synthesis. Lipid droplets accumulate within glioblastoma cells, serving as reservoirs of energy and metabolic intermediates that support tumor growth and survival under nutrient-deprived conditions. Dysregulated expression of lipogenic enzymes, fatty acid transporters, and oncogenic signaling pathways, such as AMPK and mTOR, contribute to lipid metabolic reprogramming in glioblastoma, promoting tumor aggressiveness and therapeutic resistance.

Redox Homeostasis and Oxidative Stress: Metabolic reprogramming in glioblastoma cells generates reactive oxygen species (ROS) as byproducts of aerobic metabolism, leading to oxidative stress and DNA damage. To maintain redox homeostasis and protect against oxidative damage, glioblastoma cells upregulate antioxidant defense mechanisms, including the expression of antioxidant enzymes such as superoxide dismutase (SOD) and glutathione peroxidase (GPx). Dysregulated redox signaling pathways, such as the NRF2/ARE pathway, contribute to oxidative stress resistance in glioblastoma cells, promoting tumor survival and therapeutic resistance.

Clinical Implications of Metabolic Reprogramming: Metabolic reprogramming in glioblastoma cells influences tumor aggressiveness, therapeutic response, and patient outcomes, underscoring its clinical significance as a potential therapeutic target. Elevated levels of metabolic markers such as lactate dehydrogenase (LDH), glutaminase, and fatty acid synthase within glioblastoma tumors correlate with poor prognosis and reduced overall survival in patients, highlighting the prognostic value of metabolic biomarkers. Additionally, metabolic reprogramming contributes to therapeutic resistance by promoting tumor cell survival, adaptation to the tumor microenvironment, and evasion of immune surveillance.

Therapeutic Opportunities: Targeting metabolic vulnerabilities in glioblastoma represents a promising therapeutic strategy for improving patient outcomes and overcoming treatment resistance. Therapeutic interventions aimed at disrupting glucose metabolism, glutamine metabolism, lipid metabolism, and redox homeostasis have shown promise in preclinical studies and early-phase clinical trials. Small molecule inhibitors targeting key metabolic enzymes, such as hexokinase, glutaminase, and fatty acid synthase, may offer opportunities for disrupting metabolic dependencies and sensitizing glioblastoma cells to conventional therapies.

Future Directions: Despite significant advances in our understanding of metabolic reprogramming in glioblastoma, challenges remain in translating this knowledge into effective therapeutic interventions that improve patient outcomes. Tumor heterogeneity, metabolic plasticity, and the dynamic nature of the tumor microenvironment pose formidable obstacles to successful treatment. Future research efforts aimed at elucidating the molecular mechanisms underlying metabolic reprogramming in glioblastoma, identifying novel therapeutic targets, and developing combination treatment strategies hold promise for revolutionizing the management of this devastating disease and improving patient survival and quality of life.

Conclusion: In conclusion, metabolic reprogramming emerges as a central hallmark of glioblastoma biology, fueling tumor growth, invasion, and therapeutic resistance. Understanding the intricacies of metabolic reprogramming in glioblastoma is essential for developing targeted therapeutic strategies aimed at disrupting tumor metabolism and improving patient outcomes. Further research into the molecular mechanisms and metabolic dependencies of glioblastoma holds promise for identifying novel therapeutic targets and developing innovative treatment approaches that target the metabolic vulnerabilities of this devastating disease.

Immune Evasion Mechanisms in Glioblastoma: Subverting the Host Defense

Glioblastoma, a highly aggressive primary brain tumor, employs a variety of immune evasion mechanisms to evade detection and destruction by the host immune system. The intricate interplay between glioblastoma cells and the immune microenvironment contributes to tumor immune escape, progression, and therapeutic resistance. Understanding the mechanisms underlying immune evasion in glioblastoma is crucial for developing effective immunotherapeutic strategies aimed at harnessing the immune system to target and eradicate tumor cells. In this comprehensive exploration, we delve into the diverse array of immune evasion mechanisms employed by glioblastoma, unraveling their molecular underpinnings, clinical implications, and therapeutic opportunities.

Tumor Heterogeneity and Immune Privilege: Glioblastoma exhibits intratumoral and intertumoral heterogeneity, characterized by diverse phenotypic and molecular profiles that contribute to immune evasion and therapeutic resistance. Glioblastoma cells exploit the immune-privileged environment of the central nervous system (CNS) to evade immune surveillance and establish an immunosuppressive microenvironment conducive to tumor growth and progression. The blood-brain barrier (BBB) restricts the entry of immune cells and therapeutic agents into the CNS, further exacerbating immune evasion and limiting the efficacy of immunotherapy in glioblastoma.

Immunosuppressive Signaling Pathways: Glioblastoma cells employ a variety of immunosuppressive signaling pathways to dampen anti-tumor immune responses and promote immune tolerance within the tumor microenvironment. Dysregulated expression of immune checkpoint molecules, such as programmed cell death protein 1 (PD-1), programmed death-ligand 1 (PD-L1), cytotoxic T-lymphocyte-associated protein 4 (CTLA-4), and T-cell immunoglobulin and mucin-domain containing-3 (TIM-3), inhibits T-cell activation and effector function, allowing tumor cells to evade immune recognition and destruction. Additionally, glioblastoma cells secrete immunosuppressive cytokines such as transforming growth factor-beta (TGF-β) and interleukin-10 (IL-10), which suppress effector T-cell responses and promote the expansion of regulatory T cells (Tregs) and myeloid-derived suppressor cells (MDSCs) within the tumor microenvironment.

Tumor-Associated Macrophages and Myeloid-Derived Suppressor Cells: Tumor-associated macrophages (TAMs) and myeloid-derived suppressor cells (MDSCs) play a central role in immune evasion and tumor progression in glioblastoma. TAMs exhibit an immunosuppressive M2-like phenotype, characterized by the secretion of anti-inflammatory cytokines and growth factors that promote tumor growth, invasion, and angiogenesis. MDSCs suppress anti-tumor immune responses through various mechanisms, including the production of immunosuppressive factors such as arginase-1 (Arg1) and inducible nitric oxide synthase (iNOS), inhibition of T-cell proliferation and activation, and induction of T-cell apoptosis.

Tumor-Induced Immunomodulation: Glioblastoma cells modulate the immune microenvironment through various mechanisms to promote tumor immune escape and therapeutic resistance. Tumor-derived extracellular vesicles (EVs), including exosomes and microvesicles, shuttle immunosuppressive molecules such as PD-L1, TGF-β, and miRNAs to neighboring immune cells, promoting immune evasion and tumor progression. Additionally, metabolic reprogramming in glioblastoma cells alters the composition and function of immune cells within the tumor microenvironment, leading to immune dysfunction and therapeutic resistance.

Clinical Implications and Therapeutic Opportunities: Immune evasion mechanisms in glioblastoma pose significant challenges to immunotherapy and limit the efficacy of current treatment modalities. Understanding the molecular underpinnings of immune evasion in glioblastoma is essential for developing effective immunotherapeutic strategies aimed at overcoming immune resistance and improving patient outcomes. Therapeutic interventions targeting immune checkpoint molecules, such as PD-1/PD-L1 and CTLA-4, have shown promise in preclinical studies and early-phase clinical trials, offering opportunities for restoring anti-tumor immune responses and enhancing therapeutic efficacy in glioblastoma.

Future Directions: Despite significant advances in our understanding of immune evasion mechanisms in glioblastoma, challenges remain in translating this knowledge into effective therapeutic interventions that improve patient outcomes. Tumor heterogeneity, immune cell plasticity, and the dynamic nature of the tumor microenvironment pose formidable obstacles to successful treatment. Future research efforts aimed at elucidating the molecular mechanisms underlying immune evasion in glioblastoma, identifying novel therapeutic targets, and developing combination treatment strategies hold promise for revolutionizing the management of this devastating disease and improving patient survival and quality of life.

Conclusion: In conclusion, immune evasion mechanisms play a central role in glioblastoma progression, therapeutic resistance, and poor clinical outcomes. Understanding the complex interplay between glioblastoma cells and the immune microenvironment is essential for developing effective immunotherapeutic strategies aimed at overcoming immune resistance and improving patient outcomes. Further research into the molecular mechanisms and therapeutic vulnerabilities of immune evasion in glioblastoma holds promise for advancing our understanding of this devastating disease and developing innovative treatment approaches that harness the power of the immune system to target and eradicate tumor cells.

CHAPTER 4: CLINICAL PRESENTATION AND SYMPTOMS

Early Symptoms of Glioblastoma: Recognizing the Initial Signs

Glioblastoma, the most aggressive primary brain tumor, often presents with insidious onset and nonspecific symptoms in its early stages, making early diagnosis challenging. However, recognizing the subtle warning signs of glioblastoma is crucial for initiating timely diagnostic evaluation and treatment, potentially improving patient outcomes. In this comprehensive exploration, we delve into the early symptoms of glioblastoma, unraveling their clinical manifestations, diagnostic significance, and implications for patient management.

1. Headaches: Persistent and severe headaches, often described as dull or throbbing in nature, represent one of the most common early symptoms of glioblastoma. These headaches may worsen over time, become more frequent, and often occur in the morning or upon awakening. Headaches associated with glioblastoma may not respond to over-the-counter pain medications and may be accompanied by other neurological symptoms.

2. Cognitive Changes: Glioblastoma can affect cognitive function in its early stages, leading to subtle changes in memory, concentration, and executive function. Patients may experience difficulty with multitasking, organizing thoughts, and completing tasks that were previously effortless. Cognitive changes may be subtle and may initially go unnoticed by patients and their caregivers.

3. Visual Disturbances: Visual disturbances, such as blurred vision, double vision (diplopia), and visual field deficits, may occur in the early stages of glioblastoma, particularly if the tumor affects regions of the brain involved in visual processing. Patients may notice difficulty reading, driving, or navigating their surroundings due to visual impairment.

4. Seizures: Seizures, particularly focal seizures affecting one part of the body, are common early symptoms of glioblastoma. Seizures may manifest as sudden jerking movements, sensory disturbances, altered consciousness, or loss of awareness. Seizures may occur spontaneously or may be triggered by specific stimuli, such as flashing lights or emotional stress.

5. Motor Weakness or Coordination Problems: Glioblastoma can cause motor weakness, loss of coordination, and difficulty with fine motor tasks in its early stages. Patients may experience weakness or numbness in one side of the body, clumsiness, and difficulty with activities such as writing, buttoning clothing, or using utensils.

6. Speech and Language Difficulties: Glioblastoma affecting regions of the brain involved in speech and language processing may lead to difficulties with speech production, comprehension, and articulation. Patients may experience slurred speech, difficulty finding words (anomia), and problems with fluency and grammar.

7. Personality Changes and Mood Disturbances: Glioblastoma can cause changes in personality, mood, and behavior in its early stages, often attributed to the tumor's effects on emotional regulation and social cognition. Patients may exhibit irritability, apathy, disinhibition, or emotional lability that is uncharacteristic of their baseline personality.

8. Nausea and Vomiting: Nausea and vomiting may occur in the early stages of glioblastoma, often attributed to increased intracranial pressure resulting from tumor growth and edema. These symptoms may be intermittent and may worsen with changes in body position, such as bending over or lying down.

9. Fatigue and Malaise: Fatigue, weakness, and generalized malaise may be early symptoms of glioblastoma, reflecting the body's systemic response to tumor growth and metabolic changes. Patients may experience profound fatigue that is not relieved by rest and may interfere with daily activities and quality of life.

10. Changes in Appetite and Weight Loss: Glioblastoma can affect appetite and eating habits in its early stages, leading to changes in appetite, taste preferences, and weight loss. Patients may experience loss of appetite, early satiety, or aversion to certain foods, leading to unintended weight loss and nutritional deficiencies.

Conclusion: Early recognition of the subtle warning signs of glioblastoma is essential for initiating timely diagnostic evaluation and treatment, potentially improving patient outcomes. Healthcare providers should maintain a high index of suspicion for glioblastoma in patients presenting with nonspecific neurological symptoms, particularly those that are progressive, persistent, or unexplained. Prompt referral to a neurologist or neurosurgeon for further evaluation and neuroimaging is warranted in patients with suspected glioblastoma, allowing for timely diagnosis and intervention. Early detection and intervention may offer the best chance for optimizing patient outcomes and quality of life in glioblastoma.

Progression of Symptoms in Glioblastoma: Unveiling the Evolving Clinical Course

As glioblastoma progresses, the clinical manifestations experienced by patients often undergo a dynamic evolution, reflecting the relentless growth and invasive nature of the tumor within the intricate confines of the brain. Understanding the pattern of symptom progression in glioblastoma is crucial for healthcare providers to anticipate the changing needs of patients, optimize symptom management, and facilitate timely adjustments in treatment strategies. In this comprehensive exploration, we delve into the progression of symptoms in glioblastoma, unraveling the evolving clinical course and its implications for patient care.

1. **Intensification of Headaches:** Headaches, a hallmark symptom of glioblastoma, often intensify and become more frequent as the tumor grows and exerts increasing pressure on surrounding brain tissue. Patients may experience severe, persistent headaches that are refractory to conventional pain medications and may worsen with changes in body position or physical activity. Headaches may become incapacitating and significantly impair the patient's quality of life.

2. **Neurological Deficits:** As glioblastoma infiltrates and disrupts normal brain function, patients may develop progressive neurological deficits corresponding to the affected areas of the brain. Motor weakness, sensory disturbances, and coordination problems may worsen over time, leading to functional impairment and loss of independence. Patients may experience difficulty with activities of daily living, such as walking, dressing, and feeding themselves.

3. **Seizure Burden:** Seizures, a common complication of glioblastoma, may increase in frequency and severity as the tumor progresses. Patients may experience more frequent and prolonged seizures, which may be refractory to antiepileptic medications and require additional interventions, such as seizure monitoring and adjustment of medication dosages. Seizures may become increasingly debilitating and impact the patient's ability to perform daily activities.

4. **Cognitive Decline:** Glioblastoma-related cognitive deficits, including memory impairment, executive dysfunction, and language difficulties, may progress over time as the

tumor disrupts critical brain regions involved in cognitive function. Patients may experience worsening cognitive decline, affecting their ability to communicate, make decisions, and perform complex tasks. Cognitive deficits may have profound implications for the patient's overall functioning and quality of life.

5. Visual Impairment: Visual disturbances, such as blurred vision, visual field deficits, and diplopia, may worsen as glioblastoma infiltrates regions of the brain involved in visual processing. Patients may experience progressive visual impairment, leading to difficulty reading, navigating their surroundings, and performing activities that require visual acuity. Visual deficits may significantly impact the patient's independence and quality of life.

6. Personality Changes and Psychiatric Symptoms: Glioblastoma-related alterations in personality, mood, and behavior may escalate as the tumor progresses and affects regions of the brain involved in emotional regulation and social cognition. Patients may exhibit worsening irritability, agitation, apathy, or disinhibition, which may be distressing for both the patient and their caregivers. Psychiatric symptoms may require multidisciplinary interventions, including psychosocial support and pharmacological management.

7. Functional Decline and Dependency: As glioblastoma advances, patients may experience progressive functional decline and increasing dependency on caregivers for assistance with activities of daily living. Motor deficits, cognitive impairment, and other neurological symptoms may limit the patient's ability to perform basic self-care tasks, necessitating ongoing support and assistance from family members or healthcare providers.

8. Decline in Performance Status: Glioblastoma-related symptoms and complications may lead to a decline in performance status, as reflected by worsening scores on performance status scales such as the Karnofsky Performance

Status (KPS) or Eastern Cooperative Oncology Group (ECOG) performance status. Patients may experience increasing fatigue, weakness, and overall debility, impacting their ability to tolerate treatment and participate in daily activities.

Conclusion: The progression of symptoms in glioblastoma is characterized by a dynamic evolution reflecting the aggressive nature of the tumor and its impact on brain function and neurological integrity. Healthcare providers should be vigilant in monitoring patients for changes in symptoms and functional status, anticipating the evolving needs of patients and providing timely interventions to optimize symptom management and quality of life. Multidisciplinary care teams, including neurologists, neurosurgeons, oncologists, palliative care specialists, and allied healthcare professionals, play a crucial role in supporting patients and their families throughout the continuum of glioblastoma care. By understanding the pattern of symptom progression in glioblastoma and addressing the evolving clinical course with tailored interventions, healthcare providers can enhance the quality of care and improve outcomes for patients living with this devastating disease.

Location-Specific Symptoms in Glioblastoma: Deciphering the Manifestations

Glioblastoma, with its propensity to infiltrate various regions of the brain, often presents with location-specific symptoms that reflect the anatomical structures affected by tumor growth. Recognizing these symptoms is essential for healthcare providers to localize the tumor and tailor treatment strategies accordingly. In this comprehensive exploration, we delve into the manifestations of glioblastoma based on its location within the brain, unraveling the diverse array of location-specific symptoms and their clinical significance.

1. Frontal Lobe:

- **Personality Changes and Behavioral Disturbances:**

Glioblastoma in the frontal lobe may manifest as alterations in personality, mood swings, disinhibition, and executive dysfunction.

- **Motor Weakness and Coordination Problems:** Patients may experience weakness or paralysis of contralateral limbs, along with difficulties with coordination and fine motor tasks.

2. Parietal Lobe:

- **Sensory Deficits:** Glioblastoma in the parietal lobe may lead to sensory disturbances, including numbness, tingling, and loss of sensation on the contralateral side of the body.
- **Visual-Spatial Impairment:** Patients may experience difficulty with spatial orientation, navigation, and visual-spatial processing.

3. Temporal Lobe:

- **Memory Impairment:** Glioblastoma in the temporal lobe may result in memory deficits, including difficulty with encoding and retrieving new information (anterograde amnesia) and recalling past events (retrograde amnesia).
- **Auditory Hallucinations:** Patients may experience auditory hallucinations, such as hearing voices or sounds, due to involvement of the auditory cortex.

4. Occipital Lobe:

- **Visual Disturbances:** Glioblastoma in the occipital lobe may cause visual disturbances, including visual field deficits, blurry vision, and visual hallucinations.
- **Impaired Visual Processing:** Patients may have difficulty recognizing objects, faces, or colors due to disruption of visual processing pathways.

5. Brainstem:

- **Cranial Nerve Dysfunction:** Glioblastoma involving

the brainstem may lead to cranial nerve deficits, such as diplopia (CN III, IV, VI), facial weakness (CN VII), dysphagia (CN IX, X, XII), and dysarthria (CN IX, X, XII).
- **Motor and Sensory Deficits:** Patients may experience weakness, numbness, or paralysis of limbs, along with difficulties with balance and coordination.

6. Cerebellum:

- **Ataxia:** Glioblastoma in the cerebellum may cause ataxia, characterized by unsteady gait, coordination problems, and difficulties with fine motor tasks.
- **Nystagmus:** Patients may experience involuntary eye movements, such as nystagmus, due to disruption of cerebellar pathways.

7. Corpus Callosum:

- **Cognitive Impairment:** Glioblastoma involving the corpus callosum may lead to cognitive deficits, including impaired attention, processing speed, and interhemispheric communication.
- **Apraxia:** Patients may have difficulty performing skilled motor movements, such as dressing or using utensils, due to disruption of callosal connections.

8. Basal Ganglia:

- **Movement Disorders:** Glioblastoma in the basal ganglia may manifest as movement disorders, including chorea, dystonia, and bradykinesia, due to disruption of motor control circuits.
- **Personality Changes:** Patients may exhibit alterations in mood, behavior, and motivation, reflecting dysfunction of the limbic system.

Conclusion: Location-specific symptoms in glioblastoma provide valuable insights into the anatomical localization of the tumor and its impact on brain function and neurological integrity. Healthcare providers should carefully evaluate patients for these symptoms to localize the tumor and guide treatment decisions. Multimodal imaging techniques, such as MRI and PET scans, play a crucial role in delineating the anatomical extent of the tumor and identifying location-specific manifestations. By recognizing and addressing location-specific symptoms, healthcare providers can optimize patient care and improve outcomes for individuals living with glioblastoma.

Neurological Manifestations of Glioblastoma: Unveiling the Complex Neurological Landscape

Glioblastoma, with its invasive nature and propensity to infiltrate various regions of the brain, manifests with a diverse array of neurological symptoms that reflect the complex interplay between tumor growth and disruption of normal brain function. Recognizing these neurological manifestations is essential for healthcare providers to assess disease progression, tailor treatment strategies, and optimize symptom management. In this comprehensive exploration, we delve into the neurological manifestations of glioblastoma, unraveling the multifaceted clinical landscape and its implications for patient care.

1. **Motor Deficits:**
   - **Weakness and Paralysis:** Glioblastoma can lead to weakness or paralysis of limbs on one side of the body (hemiparesis or hemiplegia), reflecting the involvement of motor pathways in the brain.
   - **Coordination Problems:** Patients may experience difficulties with coordination, balance, and fine motor tasks due to disruption of cerebellar or basal ganglia function.
2. **Sensory Disturbances:**
   - **Numbness and Tingling:** Glioblastoma may cause

sensory deficits, such as numbness, tingling, or loss of sensation, typically affecting one side of the body.
- **Paresthesias:** Patients may experience abnormal sensations, such as burning, prickling, or crawling sensations, due to disruption of sensory pathways.

3. Seizures:
- **Focal Seizures:** Glioblastoma often presents with focal seizures originating from the area of the brain affected by tumor growth, manifesting as motor, sensory, or psychic symptoms depending on the location of the seizure focus.
- **Generalized Seizures:** Seizures may generalize and involve both hemispheres of the brain, leading to loss of consciousness, convulsions, and postictal confusion.

4. Cognitive Dysfunction:
- **Memory Impairment:** Glioblastoma-related cognitive deficits may include difficulty with short-term memory, encoding and retrieval of new information, and recalling past events.
- **Executive Dysfunction:** Patients may experience difficulties with planning, organization, problem-solving, and decision-making, reflecting impairment of frontal lobe function.

5. Language and Speech Disturbances:
- **Aphasia:** Glioblastoma affecting language areas in the dominant hemisphere may lead to aphasia, characterized by difficulty with language comprehension, expression, or both.
- **Dysarthria:** Patients may exhibit slurred or impaired speech articulation due to weakness or dysfunction of the muscles involved in speech production.

6. Visual Impairment:

- **Visual Field Deficits:** Glioblastoma may cause visual field defects, such as hemianopsia or quadrantanopsia, due to compression or infiltration of the optic pathways.
- **Visual Disturbances:** Patients may experience blurry vision, double vision (diplopia), photophobia, or visual hallucinations due to disruption of visual processing pathways.

7. **Personality and Behavioral Changes:**
   - **Emotional Lability:** Glioblastoma-related alterations in personality and behavior may manifest as emotional lability, mood swings, irritability, apathy, or disinhibition.
   - **Psychiatric Symptoms:** Patients may exhibit symptoms of depression, anxiety, psychosis, or mania, reflecting the tumor's impact on emotional regulation and social cognition.

8. **Headache and Intracranial Pressure Symptoms:**
   - **Persistent Headaches:** Glioblastoma-related headaches may be severe, persistent, and worsen over time, often accompanied by nausea, vomiting, and photophobia.
   - **Increased Intracranial Pressure:** Patients may experience symptoms of increased intracranial pressure, such as papilledema, altered consciousness, and signs of herniation syndromes (e.g., cranial nerve palsies, hemiparesis).

Conclusion: The neurological manifestations of glioblastoma encompass a broad spectrum of symptoms reflecting the intricate interplay between tumor growth and disruption of normal brain function. Healthcare providers should carefully evaluate patients for these neurological symptoms to assess disease progression, guide treatment decisions, and optimize symptom management. Multimodal imaging techniques, such as MRI and PET scans, play a crucial role in delineating the anatomical extent of the tumor and identifying associated neurological deficits. By recognizing and addressing the diverse neurological manifestations of glioblastoma, healthcare providers can improve outcomes and enhance the quality of life for individuals living with this devastating disease.

Cognitive and Behavioral Changes in Glioblastoma: Understanding the Neuropsychological Landscape

Glioblastoma, with its pervasive infiltration of the brain, often manifests with cognitive and behavioral changes that significantly impact the quality of life of affected individuals. These alterations in cognition and behavior arise from the intricate interplay between tumor growth, disruption of neural circuits, and the tumor microenvironment. Recognizing and addressing these changes is essential for healthcare providers to optimize patient care and support patients and their families throughout the disease trajectory. In this comprehensive exploration, we delve into the cognitive and behavioral changes observed in glioblastoma, unraveling the complex neuropsychological landscape and its implications for patient management.

1. **Memory Impairment:**
   - **Short-Term Memory Loss:** Glioblastoma can lead to deficits in short-term memory, affecting the ability to retain and recall recent events or information.
   - **Long-Term Memory Impairment:** Patients may experience difficulties with retrieving memories of past events, affecting autobiographical memory and historical knowledge.
2. **Executive Dysfunction:**
   - **Planning and Organization:** Glioblastoma-related cognitive changes may impair the ability to plan

and organize tasks, leading to difficulties with time management and task completion.
- **Problem-Solving:** Patients may struggle with problem-solving and decision-making, finding it challenging to generate and evaluate alternative solutions.

3. Attention and Concentration:
- **Sustained Attention:** Glioblastoma can impair sustained attention, making it difficult for patients to maintain focus and concentration over prolonged periods.
- **Selective Attention:** Patients may have difficulty filtering out irrelevant information and focusing on relevant stimuli, affecting their ability to prioritize tasks and ignore distractions.

4. Language and Communication:
- **Expressive Language Deficits:** Glioblastoma may impair expressive language abilities, leading to difficulties with word finding, sentence construction, and articulation.
- **Receptive Language Deficits:** Patients may have difficulty understanding spoken or written language, affecting comprehension and communication with others.

5. Visuospatial Skills:
- **Spatial Awareness:** Glioblastoma-related cognitive changes may impair spatial awareness and navigation abilities, leading to difficulties with orientation and wayfinding.
- **Visuoconstructional Skills:** Patients may struggle with tasks that require the manipulation and integration of visual-spatial information, such as drawing or assembling objects.

6. Emotional Regulation:

- **Affective Lability:** Glioblastoma can lead to fluctuations in mood and emotional expression, characterized by rapid shifts between euphoria and sadness, irritability, or emotional flatness.
- **Emotional Insight:** Patients may exhibit reduced insight into their emotional experiences, finding it challenging to identify and regulate their feelings effectively.

7. Behavioral Changes:

- **Disinhibition:** Glioblastoma-related alterations in frontal lobe function may lead to disinhibited behavior, characterized by impulsivity, poor judgment, and social indiscretion.
- **Apathy:** Patients may experience reduced motivation, initiative, and interest in activities they previously enjoyed, leading to withdrawal and social isolation.

8. Psychiatric Symptoms:

- **Depression and Anxiety:** Glioblastoma can precipitate symptoms of depression and anxiety, including persistent sadness, worry, fatigue, and sleep disturbances.
- **Psychotic Symptoms:** Patients may experience hallucinations or delusions, such as auditory hallucinations or paranoid ideation, reflecting the tumor's impact on neural circuits involved in perception and reality testing.

Conclusion: Cognitive and behavioral changes in glioblastoma encompass a broad spectrum of symptoms that significantly impact the lives of affected individuals and their families. Healthcare providers should be vigilant in recognizing these changes and implementing appropriate interventions to support patients throughout the disease trajectory. Multidisciplinary care teams, including neurologists, neuropsychologists, psychiatrists, and social workers, play a crucial role in assessing and managing cognitive and behavioral symptoms in glioblastoma patients. By addressing the complex neuropsychological landscape of glioblastoma, healthcare providers can improve patient outcomes and enhance the quality of life for individuals living with this devastating disease.

Diagnostic Challenges and Differential Diagnosis in Glioblastoma: Navigating the Complex Diagnostic Pathway

The diagnosis of glioblastoma presents numerous challenges due to its varied clinical presentations, nonspecific symptoms, and overlapping features with other brain pathologies. Distinguishing glioblastoma from other brain tumors and non-neoplastic conditions requires a comprehensive diagnostic approach incorporating clinical, radiological, histopathological, and molecular assessments. In this comprehensive exploration, we delve into the diagnostic challenges and differential diagnosis of glioblastoma, unraveling the complexities of the diagnostic pathway and its implications for patient management.

1. Clinical Presentation:

- **Nonspecific Symptoms:** Glioblastoma often presents with nonspecific symptoms, such as headache, cognitive changes, and focal neurological deficits, which can mimic other neurological disorders.
- **Insidious Onset:** The gradual onset and progression of symptoms in glioblastoma may lead to delayed diagnosis, as patients may attribute their symptoms to other causes or dismiss them as part of the normal aging process.

2. Radiological Findings:

- **Imaging Features:** Glioblastoma typically appears as an infiltrative mass with irregular borders and heterogeneous enhancement on contrast-enhanced MRI, making it challenging to differentiate from other brain tumors, such as metastases or lymphomas.
- **Pseudoprogression:** Treatment-related changes, including radiation necrosis and pseudoprogression, can mimic tumor progression on imaging studies, necessitating careful interpretation and follow-up imaging assessments.

3. **Histopathological Evaluation:**
   - **Tumor Biopsy:** Definitive diagnosis of glioblastoma requires histopathological examination of tissue obtained via surgical biopsy or resection, which may be associated with risks and complications.
   - **Histological Variants:** Glioblastoma encompasses various histological variants, including giant cell glioblastoma, gliosarcoma, and epithelioid glioblastoma, each with distinct morphological features and prognostic implications.

4. **Molecular Profiling:**
   - **IDH Mutation Status:** The presence of mutations in the isocitrate dehydrogenase (IDH) genes distinguishes IDH-mutant glioblastoma from IDH-wildtype glioblastoma and is associated with differences in tumor biology and patient prognosis.
   - **MGMT Promoter Methylation:** MGMT promoter methylation status predicts response to alkylating chemotherapy agents, such as temozolomide, and is a prognostic biomarker in glioblastoma.

5. **Differential Diagnosis:**
   - **Metastatic Brain Tumors:** Metastases to the brain, particularly from lung, breast, or melanoma primaries,

can mimic glioblastoma on imaging studies and may require tissue biopsy for definitive diagnosis.
- **Primary Central Nervous System Lymphoma (PCNSL):** PCNSL shares radiological and histological features with glioblastoma and may require immunohistochemical and molecular analyses for accurate diagnosis.
- **Infectious and Inflammatory Disorders:** Non-neoplastic conditions, such as cerebral abscesses, demyelinating diseases, and autoimmune encephalitis, may present with symptoms and imaging findings overlapping with glioblastoma, necessitating thorough clinical evaluation and ancillary testing.

6. Multidisciplinary Evaluation:

- **Tumor Board Review:** A multidisciplinary approach involving neurosurgeons, neuro-oncologists, neuroradiologists, neuropathologists, and radiation oncologists is essential for accurate diagnosis and treatment planning in glioblastoma.
- **Integration of Clinical and Radiological Data:** Clinical correlation with radiological findings, histopathological assessment, and molecular profiling is critical for establishing an accurate diagnosis and guiding personalized treatment decisions.

Conclusion: The diagnosis of glioblastoma poses significant challenges due to its varied clinical presentations, radiological features, and histopathological characteristics. Healthcare providers must adopt a comprehensive diagnostic approach incorporating clinical evaluation, neuroimaging, tissue biopsy, and molecular profiling to differentiate glioblastoma from other brain tumors and non-neoplastic conditions accurately. By navigating the complexities of the diagnostic pathway and leveraging multidisciplinary expertise, healthcare providers can ensure timely diagnosis and appropriate management of patients with glioblastoma, ultimately improving patient outcomes and quality of life.

CHAPTER 5: DIAGNOSTIC MODALITIES

Neuroimaging Techniques in Glioblastoma: Unraveling the Intricacies of MRI, CT, and PET

Neuroimaging plays a pivotal role in the diagnosis, characterization, treatment planning, and monitoring of glioblastoma, providing invaluable insights into the anatomical, functional, and metabolic aspects of the tumor and its surrounding brain tissue. Magnetic resonance imaging (MRI), computed tomography (CT), and positron emission tomography (PET) are the primary imaging modalities employed in the management of glioblastoma, each offering unique advantages and applications in clinical practice. In this comprehensive exploration, we delve into the intricacies of MRI, CT, and PET imaging techniques in glioblastoma, elucidating their principles, methodologies, and clinical utility in the management of this devastating disease.

1. Magnetic Resonance Imaging (MRI): Magnetic resonance imaging (MRI) is the cornerstone of neuroimaging in glioblastoma, offering unparalleled spatial resolution, tissue contrast, and multiplanar imaging capabilities. MRI utilizes strong magnetic fields and radiofrequency pulses to generate detailed images of the brain, allowing for the visualization of tumor morphology, extent of infiltration, and associated changes in surrounding brain tissue. Key MRI sequences used in the evaluation of glioblastoma include:

- **T1-weighted Imaging:** T1-weighted images provide excellent anatomical detail and contrast between gray and white matter, allowing for the visualization of tumor location, size, and morphology. Glioblastomas typically appear hypointense on T1-weighted images.
- **T2-weighted Imaging:** T2-weighted images highlight abnormalities in tissue water content, providing insights into tumor edema, infiltration, and mass effect on adjacent structures. Glioblastomas often exhibit hyperintensity on T2-weighted images due to surrounding edema.
- **Fluid-attenuated Inversion Recovery (FLAIR):** FLAIR imaging suppresses the signal from cerebrospinal fluid (CSF), enhancing the visualization of peritumoral edema and tumor margins. FLAIR sequences are particularly useful for assessing tumor infiltration into surrounding brain tissue.
- **Gadolinium-enhanced Imaging:** Gadolinium-based contrast agents are administered intravenously to highlight areas of blood-brain barrier disruption and tumor enhancement. Gadolinium-enhanced T1-weighted images facilitate the detection of glioblastoma and differentiation from surrounding brain tissue.

2. Computed Tomography (CT): Computed tomography (CT) provides rapid and readily available imaging of the brain, offering valuable information about tumor location, size, density, and associated changes. CT imaging utilizes X-rays and computerized reconstruction techniques to generate cross-sectional images of the brain, allowing for the detection and characterization of glioblastoma. Key features of CT imaging in glioblastoma include:

- **Contrast-enhanced CT:** Intravenous administration of

iodinated contrast agents enables the visualization of tumor enhancement, necrosis, and associated vascular abnormalities. Contrast-enhanced CT scans provide complementary information to MRI in the evaluation of glioblastoma.

- **CT Angiography (CTA):** CTA allows for the visualization of the intracranial vasculature and assessment of tumor vascularity, providing insights into tumor perfusion, angiogenesis, and vascular encasement.
- **Perfusion CT:** Perfusion CT techniques measure cerebral blood flow and blood volume within the tumor and surrounding brain tissue, aiding in the assessment of tumor vascularity and response to therapy.

3. Positron Emission Tomography (PET): Positron emission tomography (PET) imaging offers functional and metabolic information about glioblastoma, complementing structural imaging modalities such as MRI and CT. PET imaging utilizes radiotracer agents, such as 18F-fluorodeoxyglucose (FDG) or 18F-fluoromisonidazole (FMISO), to visualize glucose metabolism, hypoxia, and cellular proliferation within the tumor. Key applications of PET imaging in glioblastoma include:

- **18F-FDG PET:** FDG-PET assesses glucose metabolism within the tumor and surrounding brain tissue, providing insights into tumor aggressiveness, proliferation, and response to therapy. Glioblastomas typically exhibit increased FDG uptake compared to normal brain tissue.
- **18F-FMISO PET:** FMISO-PET detects hypoxia within the tumor microenvironment, which is associated with treatment resistance, tumor recurrence, and poor prognosis in glioblastoma. FMISO-PET imaging may help identify hypoxic regions for targeted therapy and radiation dose escalation.

Conclusion: Neuroimaging techniques, including MRI, CT, and PET, play a crucial role in the diagnosis, characterization, and management of glioblastoma, offering valuable insights into tumor morphology, vascularity, metabolism, and treatment response. Integration of multimodal imaging data enables comprehensive evaluation of glioblastoma and guides personalized treatment strategies tailored to the individual patient's disease characteristics. By leveraging the strengths of MRI, CT, and PET imaging modalities, healthcare providers can optimize patient care, improve treatment outcomes, and enhance the quality of life for individuals living with glioblastoma.

Histopathological Evaluation in Glioblastoma: Unveiling the Tumor's Cellular Landscape

Histopathological evaluation serves as the cornerstone of diagnosis and characterization in glioblastoma, providing crucial insights into the tumor's cellular composition, histological features, and molecular alterations. Glioblastoma, characterized by its aggressive behavior and complex genetic profile, poses unique challenges in histopathological assessment, necessitating a comprehensive approach integrating traditional histology, immunohistochemistry, and molecular pathology techniques. In this comprehensive exploration, we delve into the intricacies of histopathological evaluation in glioblastoma, unraveling the tumor's cellular landscape and its implications for diagnosis, prognosis, and therapeutic decision-making.

1. Tissue Acquisition and Processing:
- **Surgical Biopsy or Resection:** Definitive diagnosis of glioblastoma requires the acquisition of tissue specimens via surgical biopsy or resection, guided by neuroimaging and intraoperative navigation techniques.

- **Frozen Section Analysis:** Intraoperative frozen section analysis enables rapid assessment of tissue specimens for diagnostic confirmation and surgical guidance, facilitating real-time decision-making during surgery.

2. **Hematoxylin and Eosin (H&E) Staining:**
   - **Cellular Morphology:** Hematoxylin and eosin (H&E) staining provides detailed visualization of cellular morphology, nuclear characteristics, and tissue architecture, allowing for the identification of key histological features of glioblastoma.
   - **Key Histological Features:** Glioblastoma is characterized by cellular pleomorphism, nuclear atypia, microvascular proliferation, pseudopalisading necrosis, and infiltrative growth pattern on H&E-stained sections.

3. **Immunohistochemistry (IHC):**
   - **Biomarker Expression:** Immunohistochemistry (IHC) enables the detection of specific protein biomarkers expressed in glioblastoma, providing insights into tumor classification, differentiation, and molecular subtyping.
   - **Key Immunohistochemical Markers:** IHC markers commonly used in glioblastoma include glial fibrillary acidic protein (GFAP), Ki-67 proliferation index, p53, EGFR amplification, IDH mutation status, and MGMT promoter methylation.

4. **Molecular Pathology Techniques:**
   - **Next-Generation Sequencing (NGS):** Molecular profiling of glioblastoma using next-generation sequencing (NGS) techniques allows for the detection of somatic mutations, copy number alterations, and gene expression profiles, providing valuable prognostic and predictive information.
   - **IDH Mutation Status:** The presence of mutations

in the isocitrate dehydrogenase (IDH) genes distinguishes IDH-mutant glioblastoma from IDH-wildtype glioblastoma and is associated with differences in tumor biology and patient prognosis.
- **MGMT Promoter Methylation:** Methylation of the O6-methylguanine-DNA methyltransferase (MGMT) promoter is a predictive biomarker of response to alkylating chemotherapy agents, such as temozolomide, and is associated with improved prognosis in glioblastoma.

5. In Situ Hybridization (ISH):
- **EGFR Amplification:** In situ hybridization (ISH) techniques, such as fluorescence in situ hybridization (FISH) or chromogenic ISH, can detect amplification of the epidermal growth factor receptor (EGFR) gene, which is frequently observed in glioblastoma and may have prognostic implications.
- **IDH1 R132H Mutation:** ISH assays targeting the IDH1 R132H mutation allow for the detection of this specific mutation in glioblastoma tissue, aiding in the diagnosis of IDH-mutant glioblastoma.

6. Integration of Histopathological and Molecular Data:
- **Personalized Medicine:** Integration of histopathological and molecular data enables the development of personalized treatment strategies tailored to the individual patient's tumor characteristics and molecular profile.
- **Prognostic Stratification:** Histopathological and molecular features of glioblastoma provide valuable prognostic information, guiding therapeutic decision-making and risk stratification for patients.

Conclusion: Histopathological evaluation serves as a fundamental component of diagnosis and characterization in glioblastoma, providing essential insights into the tumor's cellular composition, histological features, and molecular alterations. Integration of traditional histology, immunohistochemistry, and molecular pathology techniques enables comprehensive assessment of glioblastoma, guiding therapeutic decision-making and prognostic stratification. By unraveling the tumor's cellular landscape through histopathological evaluation, healthcare providers can optimize patient care, improve treatment outcomes, and advance our understanding of this complex and devastating disease.

Exploring the Molecular Landscape of Glioblastoma: Insights from Molecular Biomarkers

Glioblastoma, characterized by its aggressive behavior and heterogeneous nature, exhibits a complex molecular landscape that underlies its pathogenesis, progression, and treatment response. Molecular biomarkers play a pivotal role in deciphering the molecular intricacies of glioblastoma, providing valuable insights into tumor classification, prognosis, therapeutic targeting, and personalized treatment strategies. In this comprehensive exploration, we delve into the diverse array of molecular biomarkers in glioblastoma, unraveling their significance, clinical implications, and potential for improving patient outcomes.

1. Isocitrate Dehydrogenase (IDH) Mutation:

- **IDH Mutant Glioblastoma:** Mutations in the isocitrate dehydrogenase (IDH) genes, particularly IDH1 and IDH2, are prevalent in lower-grade gliomas but rare in primary glioblastoma. IDH mutant glioblastomas exhibit distinct molecular and clinical characteristics, including younger age at diagnosis, better prognosis, and improved response to therapy compared to IDH wild-type glioblastomas.
- **Prognostic and Predictive Role:** IDH mutation status serves as a prognostic biomarker in glioblastoma, with

IDH mutant tumors associated with longer overall survival and progression-free survival. Additionally, IDH mutation status predicts response to targeted therapies and guides treatment decisions in clinical practice.

2. O6-Methylguanine-DNA Methyltransferase (MGMT) Promoter Methylation:

- **MGMT Promoter Methylation:** Methylation of the O6-methylguanine-DNA methyltransferase (MGMT) promoter is associated with silencing of the MGMT gene and reduced expression of the MGMT protein, leading to increased sensitivity to alkylating chemotherapy agents, such as temozolomide.
- **Predictive Biomarker:** MGMT promoter methylation status serves as a predictive biomarker of response to temozolomide-based chemotherapy in glioblastoma, with methylated tumors showing improved therapeutic efficacy and prolonged survival compared to unmethylated tumors.
- **Clinical Implications:** Assessment of MGMT promoter methylation status guides treatment decisions and therapeutic strategies in glioblastoma, informing the selection of patients who are most likely to benefit from temozolomide chemotherapy.

3. Epidermal Growth Factor Receptor (EGFR) Amplification:

- **EGFR Alterations:** Epidermal growth factor receptor (EGFR) alterations, including gene amplification, overexpression, and mutation, are frequently observed in glioblastoma and are associated with tumor aggressiveness, resistance to therapy, and poor prognosis.
- **Therapeutic Target:** EGFR amplification and overexpression represent potential therapeutic targets in glioblastoma, with targeted inhibitors and

monoclonal antibodies under investigation in clinical trials.
- **Diagnostic and Prognostic Significance:** Detection of EGFR amplification by molecular techniques, such as fluorescence in situ hybridization (FISH) or chromogenic in situ hybridization (CISH), provides diagnostic and prognostic information in glioblastoma, guiding treatment decisions and risk stratification for patients.

4. Phosphatase and Tensin Homolog (PTEN) Loss:
- **PTEN Alterations:** Loss of function mutations or deletions in the phosphatase and tensin homolog (PTEN) gene are frequent in glioblastoma and are associated with activation of the PI3K/AKT/mTOR signaling pathway, tumor growth, and resistance to therapy.
- **Therapeutic Implications:** PTEN loss represents a potential therapeutic target in glioblastoma, with inhibitors of the PI3K/AKT/mTOR pathway under investigation in preclinical and clinical studies.
- **Prognostic Marker:** PTEN loss serves as a prognostic marker in glioblastoma, with PTEN-deficient tumors associated with worse outcomes and shorter survival compared to PTEN-intact tumors.

5. Tumor Protein p53 (TP53) Mutation:
- **TP53 Alterations:** Mutations in the tumor protein p53 (TP53) gene are common in glioblastoma and are associated with genomic instability, aberrant cell cycle regulation, and resistance to therapy.
- **Prognostic Significance:** TP53 mutation status serves as a prognostic marker in glioblastoma, with TP53 mutant tumors associated with poorer outcomes and shorter survival compared to TP53 wild-type tumors.
- **Therapeutic Considerations:** Targeting the p53

pathway represents a potential therapeutic strategy in glioblastoma, with small molecule inhibitors and gene therapy approaches under investigation in preclinical and clinical studies.

Conclusion: Molecular biomarkers play a crucial role in unraveling the complex molecular landscape of glioblastoma and guiding personalized treatment strategies tailored to the individual patient's tumor characteristics. Integration of molecular biomarkers into clinical practice enables risk stratification, prognostic assessment, therapeutic targeting, and optimization of patient outcomes in glioblastoma. By leveraging the insights provided by molecular biomarkers, healthcare providers can advance our understanding of glioblastoma biology and improve treatment approaches for this devastating disease.

Unraveling the Intricacies of Liquid Biopsy and Circulating Tumor DNA in Glioblastoma: A Paradigm Shift in Cancer Diagnostics

Glioblastoma, with its aggressive nature and infiltrative behavior, poses significant challenges for diagnosis, treatment monitoring, and prognostication. Traditional tissue biopsy techniques, while informative, are invasive, associated with risks, and may not capture the dynamic molecular landscape of the tumor. Liquid biopsy, a minimally invasive approach for detecting circulating tumor DNA (ctDNA) and other biomarkers in peripheral blood or cerebrospinal fluid (CSF), offers a promising alternative for non-invasive molecular profiling and monitoring in glioblastoma. In this comprehensive exploration, we delve into the evolving role of liquid biopsy and ctDNA analysis in glioblastoma, unraveling their potential applications, clinical utility, and implications for patient care.

1. Principles of Liquid Biopsy: Liquid biopsy harnesses the concept of "tumor shedding," where cancer cells release fragments of DNA, RNA, proteins, and other biomolecules into the bloodstream or CSF. ctDNA, derived from tumor cells undergoing apoptosis or necrosis, serves as a surrogate marker for the genomic alterations present in the primary tumor and metastatic lesions. Key principles of liquid biopsy in glioblastoma include:

- **Minimally Invasive:** Liquid biopsy offers a minimally invasive approach for molecular profiling and monitoring, obviating the need for repeat tissue biopsies and reducing patient discomfort and procedural risks.
- **Dynamic Sampling:** Liquid biopsy enables repeated sampling over time, allowing for longitudinal monitoring of tumor evolution, treatment response, and emergence of resistance mechanisms.
- **Comprehensive Molecular Profiling:** Liquid biopsy can capture the heterogeneity of glioblastoma by analyzing multiple biomarkers, including genetic mutations, copy number alterations, and epigenetic modifications, providing insights into tumor biology and treatment resistance.

2. **Detection Methods for ctDNA:** Various techniques have been developed for the detection and analysis of ctDNA in peripheral blood or CSF, including digital PCR, next-generation sequencing (NGS), and droplet digital PCR (ddPCR). These methods enable the sensitive and specific detection of tumor-derived mutations and genomic alterations present in ctDNA. Key detection methods for ctDNA analysis include:

- **Digital PCR:** Digital PCR techniques, such as droplet digital PCR (ddPCR) and BEAMing (beads, emulsion, amplification, and magnetics), allow for absolute quantification of mutant alleles present in ctDNA, offering high sensitivity and specificity for detecting low-frequency mutations.

- **Next-Generation Sequencing (NGS):** NGS platforms enable comprehensive profiling of ctDNA, including single nucleotide variants, insertions/deletions, copy number alterations, and structural rearrangements, providing a broader molecular landscape of the tumor.
- **Methylation-Specific PCR (MSP):** Methylation-specific PCR techniques target epigenetic alterations, such as DNA methylation patterns, in ctDNA, offering insights into tumor-specific methylation signatures and potential biomarkers for early detection and prognosis.

3. Clinical Applications of Liquid Biopsy in Glioblastoma: Liquid biopsy and ctDNA analysis hold promise for a wide range of clinical applications in glioblastoma, including:

- **Diagnosis and Prognosis:** Liquid biopsy can aid in the diagnosis and prognostication of glioblastoma by detecting tumor-specific mutations, copy number alterations, and methylation patterns in ctDNA, providing insights into tumor biology and patient outcomes.
- **Treatment Selection:** Liquid biopsy enables the identification of actionable mutations and therapeutic targets in glioblastoma, guiding treatment selection and personalized therapy options based on the molecular profile of the tumor.
- **Monitoring of Treatment Response:** Liquid biopsy allows for real-time monitoring of treatment response and disease progression in glioblastoma by tracking changes in ctDNA levels, mutation burden, and clonal evolution over time, facilitating early detection of treatment resistance and disease recurrence.
- **Detection of Minimal Residual Disease:** Liquid biopsy can detect minimal residual disease (MRD) in glioblastoma patients undergoing surgery or adjuvant

therapy, providing valuable information for post-treatment surveillance and risk stratification.

4. Challenges and Future Directions: Despite the promise of liquid biopsy in glioblastoma, several challenges and limitations remain, including:

- **Sensitivity and Specificity:** Achieving high sensitivity and specificity for ctDNA detection in the context of low tumor burden and background noise remains a challenge, requiring the development of more sensitive detection methods and analytical techniques.
- **Standardization and Validation:** Standardization of pre-analytical and analytical procedures, as well as validation of liquid biopsy assays in large-scale clinical studies, are essential for ensuring the reliability and reproducibility of results.
- **Clinical Implementation:** Integration of liquid biopsy into routine clinical practice requires overcoming logistical, regulatory, and reimbursement challenges, as well as addressing patient acceptance and healthcare provider education regarding the utility and limitations of liquid biopsy in glioblastoma management.

Conclusion: Liquid biopsy and ctDNA analysis represent a paradigm shift in cancer diagnostics, offering a non-invasive, real-time approach for molecular profiling and monitoring in glioblastoma. By providing insights into tumor biology, treatment response, and disease progression, liquid biopsy has the potential to revolutionize patient care and improve outcomes in glioblastoma. As the field continues to evolve, addressing challenges and advancing our understanding of liquid biopsy technology will be critical for realizing its full potential in glioblastoma management.

The Crucial Role of Biopsy in Glioblastoma Diagnosis:

Deciphering the Tumor's Molecular Profile

Biopsy, the surgical removal of tissue for pathological examination, plays a pivotal role in the diagnosis and characterization of glioblastoma, providing essential insights into the tumor's histopathological features, molecular profile, and genetic alterations. In the context of glioblastoma, biopsy serves as the gold standard for confirming the diagnosis, guiding treatment decisions, and informing prognostication. In this comprehensive exploration, we delve into the multifaceted role of biopsy in glioblastoma diagnosis, unraveling its significance, methodologies, and implications for patient management.

1. Confirmation of Diagnosis:

- **Definitive Histopathological Assessment:** Biopsy enables the definitive histopathological assessment of glioblastoma, allowing for the identification of key histological features, including cellular pleomorphism, microvascular proliferation, pseudopalisading necrosis, and infiltrative growth pattern, characteristic of the disease.
- **Differential Diagnosis:** Biopsy aids in the differentiation of glioblastoma from other brain tumors and non-neoplastic conditions, such as metastases, lymphomas, infectious or inflammatory lesions, demyelinating diseases, and radiation necrosis, which may present with overlapping clinical and radiological features.

2. Molecular Profiling:

- **Genetic and Molecular Analysis:** Biopsy tissue serves as a valuable source for genetic and molecular analysis, enabling the identification of specific mutations, copy number alterations, and molecular subtypes associated with glioblastoma pathogenesis, prognosis, and treatment response.

- **Personalized Medicine:** Molecular profiling of biopsy specimens guides personalized treatment strategies tailored to the individual patient's tumor characteristics, including targeted therapies, immunotherapies, and molecularly targeted agents, based on the tumor's molecular profile and actionable mutations.

3. Treatment Planning and Therapeutic Decision-Making:

- **Guidance for Treatment Selection:** Biopsy results inform therapeutic decision-making and treatment selection in glioblastoma, guiding the choice of surgical resection, adjuvant therapies, and targeted interventions based on the tumor's histopathological features, molecular profile, and prognostic markers.
- **Risk Stratification:** Biopsy-derived prognostic markers, such as IDH mutation status, MGMT promoter methylation status, and molecular subtype classification, facilitate risk stratification and prognostic assessment, guiding treatment intensity and surveillance strategies for glioblastoma patients.

4. Assessment of Tumor Heterogeneity:

- **Intratumoral Heterogeneity:** Biopsy allows for the sampling of multiple regions within the tumor, providing insights into intratumoral heterogeneity and spatial variations in histopathological features, genetic mutations, and molecular alterations, which may impact treatment response and disease progression.
- **Clonal Evolution:** Biopsy-derived molecular profiling enables the characterization of clonal evolution and the emergence of treatment-resistant subclones within the tumor, informing therapeutic strategies and surveillance protocols to mitigate the risk of recurrence and treatment failure.

5. Prognostication and Follow-up:

- **Prognostic Evaluation:** Biopsy-derived prognostic markers, including histopathological features, molecular alterations, and genetic mutations, serve as prognostic indicators for glioblastoma, informing patient counseling, treatment planning, and prognostic stratification.
- **Monitoring of Treatment Response:** Repeat biopsy may be performed during the course of treatment to assess treatment response, monitor disease progression, and detect the emergence of treatment resistance, guiding adjustments to therapeutic regimens and salvage interventions as needed.

Conclusion: Biopsy plays a central role in the diagnosis, characterization, and management of glioblastoma, providing essential insights into the tumor's histopathological features, molecular profile, and genetic alterations. By facilitating accurate diagnosis, personalized treatment selection, and prognostic assessment, biopsy contributes to improved patient outcomes and enhanced understanding of glioblastoma biology. As the field of precision medicine continues to evolve, biopsy remains an indispensable tool for unraveling the complexities of glioblastoma and advancing personalized therapeutic approaches tailored to the individual patient's tumor characteristics.

CHAPTER 6: STAGING AND PROGNOSTIC FACTORS

Deciphering Glioblastoma: Insights from WHO Classification and Grading

The World Health Organization (WHO) classification system serves as a cornerstone for the classification and grading of glioblastoma, providing a standardized framework for characterizing tumors based on histological features, molecular alterations, and clinical behavior. Glioblastoma, the most aggressive form of primary brain tumor, exhibits significant heterogeneity in its presentation, prognosis, and treatment response. In this comprehensive exploration, we delve into the intricacies of the WHO classification and grading of glioblastoma, unraveling its significance, methodologies, and implications for patient management.

1. WHO Classification of Central Nervous System Tumors:

- **Historical Evolution:** The WHO classification system for central nervous system (CNS) tumors has undergone several revisions over the years, reflecting advances in our understanding of tumor biology, molecular pathology, and diagnostic techniques.
- **Current Editions:** The most recent editions of the WHO classification system, including the 4th edition (2016) and subsequent updates, provide comprehensive guidelines for the classification and

grading of glioblastoma and other CNS tumors, incorporating histological, molecular, and clinical parameters.

2. Glioblastoma Grading:

- **Grade IV Glioma:** Glioblastoma, also known as grade IV glioma, represents the most malignant and aggressive subtype of glioma, characterized by rapid growth, diffuse infiltration into surrounding brain tissue, and poor prognosis.
- **Histological Features:** Glioblastoma is characterized by cellular pleomorphism, microvascular proliferation, pseudopalisading necrosis, and infiltrative growth pattern on histopathological examination, which distinguish it from lower-grade gliomas.

3. Molecular Subtypes of Glioblastoma:

- **IDH-Wildtype Glioblastoma:** The majority of glioblastomas (~90%) are classified as IDH-wildtype, characterized by absence of mutations in the isocitrate dehydrogenase (IDH) genes (IDH1 and IDH2) and associated with older age at diagnosis, aggressive clinical course, and poorer prognosis.
- **IDH-Mutant Glioblastoma:** A subset of glioblastomas (~10%) harbor mutations in the IDH genes, particularly IDH1 R132H, and are associated with younger age at diagnosis, distinct histological features, such as oligodendroglioma-like morphology, and improved prognosis compared to IDH-wildtype glioblastomas.

4. Molecular Biomarkers:

- **MGMT Promoter Methylation:** Methylation of the O6-methylguanine-DNA methyltransferase (MGMT) promoter is associated with improved response to alkylating chemotherapy agents, such as

temozolomide, and longer survival in glioblastoma patients, providing valuable prognostic and predictive information.
- **EGFR Amplification:** Amplification of the epidermal growth factor receptor (EGFR) gene is a common molecular alteration in glioblastoma, associated with tumor aggressiveness, resistance to therapy, and poorer prognosis.

5. Clinical Implications:
- **Treatment Strategies:** The WHO classification and grading of glioblastoma guide treatment strategies and therapeutic decisions, including surgical resection, adjuvant chemotherapy, radiation therapy, and targeted therapies, based on the tumor's molecular subtype, histological grade, and prognostic markers.
- **Prognostic Assessment:** The WHO classification system facilitates prognostic assessment and risk stratification in glioblastoma patients, informing patient counseling, treatment planning, and clinical trial eligibility based on the tumor's molecular profile and histological characteristics.

Conclusion: The WHO classification and grading system serves as a fundamental framework for the classification, grading, and prognostication of glioblastoma, integrating histological, molecular, and clinical parameters to inform diagnosis, treatment selection, and prognostic assessment. By delineating molecular subtypes, histological features, and prognostic markers, the WHO classification system enhances our understanding of glioblastoma biology and guides personalized therapeutic approaches tailored to the individual patient's tumor characteristics. As the field of glioblastoma research continues to evolve, the WHO classification system remains essential for advancing our knowledge of tumor classification and improving patient outcomes in this devastating disease.

Deciphering the Molecular Subtypes of Glioblastoma: Insights into Tumor Heterogeneity and Therapeutic Implications

Glioblastoma, characterized by its aggressive behavior and heterogeneous nature, exhibits significant variability in its molecular profile, contributing to differences in treatment response, prognosis, and patient outcomes. The identification of molecular subtypes has revolutionized our understanding of glioblastoma biology, offering insights into the underlying molecular mechanisms driving tumorigenesis, progression, and therapeutic resistance. In this comprehensive exploration, we delve into the diverse array of molecular subtypes in glioblastoma, unraveling their significance, clinical implications, and potential for guiding personalized therapeutic approaches.

1. IDH-Wildtype Glioblastoma:

- **Characteristics:** IDH-wildtype glioblastoma represents the most common molecular subtype, accounting for approximately 90% of cases, and is characterized by absence of mutations in the isocitrate dehydrogenase (IDH) genes (IDH1 and IDH2).
- **Clinical Features:** IDH-wildtype glioblastomas typically occur in older patients (>55 years), exhibit aggressive clinical behavior, and are associated with poor prognosis compared to IDH-mutant glioblastomas.
- **Molecular Alterations:** IDH-wildtype glioblastomas frequently harbor genetic alterations, such as amplification of the epidermal growth factor receptor (EGFR) gene, loss of heterozygosity (LOH) on chromosome 10q, and alterations in the tumor suppressor genes PTEN and TP53.

2. IDH-Mutant Glioblastoma:

- **Characteristics:** IDH-mutant glioblastoma represents a distinct molecular subtype, accounting for approximately 10% of cases, and is characterized by mutations in the IDH genes, particularly IDH1 R132H.
- **Clinical Features:** IDH-mutant glioblastomas typically occur in younger patients (<55 years), exhibit distinct histological features, such as oligodendroglioma-like morphology, and are associated with improved prognosis compared to IDH-wildtype glioblastomas.
- **Molecular Alterations:** IDH-mutant glioblastomas often exhibit co-occurring molecular alterations, such as loss of chromosome 1p/19q, mutations in the ATRX gene, and alterations in the TERT promoter, which contribute to their unique molecular profile and clinical behavior.

3. Proneural Subtype:

- **Characterization:** The proneural subtype is one of the molecular subtypes identified in glioblastoma based on gene expression profiling, characterized by activation of neural developmental pathways and expression of proneural markers, such as PDGFRA and OLIG2.
- **Clinical Implications:** The proneural subtype is associated with younger age at diagnosis, better response to therapy, and improved prognosis compared to other molecular subtypes, suggesting potential therapeutic vulnerabilities and targeted treatment approaches.

4. Mesenchymal Subtype:

- **Characterization:** The mesenchymal subtype represents another molecular subtype of glioblastoma, characterized by activation of mesenchymal and immune response pathways, expression of mesenchymal markers, such as CHI3L1 and CD44,

and enrichment of inflammatory and immune-related signatures.
- **Clinical Implications:** The mesenchymal subtype is associated with treatment resistance, tumor recurrence, and poor prognosis, highlighting the need for novel therapeutic strategies targeting the tumor microenvironment and immune escape mechanisms.

5. Classical Subtype:
- **Characterization:** The classical subtype is defined by activation of classical signaling pathways, such as EGFR signaling, and expression of classical markers, such as EGFR amplification and PTEN loss, associated with cell cycle dysregulation and tumor growth.
- **Clinical Implications:** The classical subtype exhibits variable clinical behavior and treatment response, with some studies suggesting a worse prognosis compared to the proneural subtype but better prognosis compared to the mesenchymal subtype.

6. Neural Subtype:
- **Characterization:** The neural subtype is characterized by expression of neuronal markers and genes involved in synaptic transmission and neuronal differentiation, reflecting a more differentiated and less aggressive phenotype.
- **Clinical Implications:** The neural subtype is associated with intermediate prognosis and clinical outcomes compared to other molecular subtypes, with potential implications for treatment selection and patient management.

Conclusion: The molecular subtyping of glioblastoma has transformed our understanding of tumor heterogeneity, providing insights into the underlying molecular mechanisms driving tumorigenesis, progression, and therapeutic resistance. By delineating distinct molecular subtypes, such as IDH-wildtype, IDH-mutant, proneural, mesenchymal, classical, and neural subtypes, researchers and clinicians can tailor personalized therapeutic approaches targeting the specific molecular vulnerabilities of each subtype, ultimately improving patient outcomes and advancing precision medicine in glioblastoma management. As the field continues to evolve, further elucidation of the molecular subtypes and their clinical implications will be essential for guiding therapeutic decision-making and optimizing patient care in this devastating disease.

Navigating Prognostic Factors in Glioblastoma: Insights into Patient Outcomes and Clinical Management

Glioblastoma, characterized by its aggressive behavior and poor prognosis, poses significant challenges for patients and clinicians alike. Prognostic factors play a crucial role in predicting patient outcomes, guiding treatment decisions, and informing clinical management strategies in glioblastoma. In this comprehensive exploration, we delve into the diverse array of prognostic factors in glioblastoma, unraveling their significance, clinical implications, and potential for guiding personalized therapeutic approaches.

1. Age:
- **Impact on Prognosis:** Age is a well-established prognostic factor in glioblastoma, with older age at diagnosis associated with poorer outcomes, shorter survival, and decreased treatment tolerance compared to younger patients.
- **Clinical Implications:** Older patients (>65 years) with glioblastoma may have comorbidities, reduced functional status, and altered treatment tolerance, necessitating personalized treatment approaches tailored to individual patient factors and preferences.

2. Karnofsky Performance Status (KPS):

- **Functional Status Assessment:** Karnofsky Performance Status (KPS) is a widely used measure of functional status and performance in cancer patients, ranging from 0 (dead) to 100 (normal, no complaints, no evidence of disease).
- **Prognostic Value:** Lower KPS scores are associated with poorer prognosis, shorter survival, and decreased treatment tolerance in glioblastoma patients, reflecting reduced functional capacity and increased disease burden.

3. Extent of Surgical Resection:

- **Impact on Survival:** The extent of surgical resection, defined as the percentage of tumor removal, is a significant prognostic factor in glioblastoma, with maximal safe resection associated with improved survival, prolonged progression-free survival, and better treatment response.
- **Clinical Considerations:** Surgical resection aims to achieve maximal tumor debulking while preserving critical neurological function, with the goal of optimizing patient outcomes and enhancing the efficacy of adjuvant therapies, such as chemotherapy and radiation therapy.

4. Molecular Biomarkers:

- **IDH Mutation Status:** Mutations in the isocitrate dehydrogenase (IDH) genes, particularly IDH1 R132H, are associated with improved prognosis, longer survival, and distinct clinical characteristics in glioblastoma patients, including younger age at diagnosis and better response to therapy.
- **MGMT Promoter Methylation:** Methylation of the O6-methylguanine-DNA methyltransferase (MGMT) promoter is predictive of response to alkylating chemotherapy agents, such as temozolomide, and

is associated with improved prognosis and longer survival in glioblastoma patients.

5. Molecular Subtypes:

- **Proneural Subtype:** The proneural molecular subtype of glioblastoma is associated with better prognosis, younger age at diagnosis, and improved response to therapy compared to other molecular subtypes, suggesting potential therapeutic vulnerabilities and targeted treatment approaches.

- **Mesenchymal Subtype:** The mesenchymal molecular subtype is associated with poorer prognosis, treatment resistance, and tumor recurrence, highlighting the need for novel therapeutic strategies targeting the tumor microenvironment and immune escape mechanisms.

6. Treatment Response:

- **Assessment of Response:** Monitoring treatment response, including radiological assessment of tumor size and volume, clinical evaluation of neurological function, and molecular profiling of residual disease, provides valuable prognostic information and guides treatment adjustments in glioblastoma patients.

- **Dynamic Treatment Strategies:** Individualized treatment approaches, incorporating serial assessment of treatment response and adaptive treatment strategies, enable optimization of patient outcomes and adjustment of therapeutic regimens based on tumor behavior and treatment response over time.

Conclusion: Prognostic factors play a critical role in predicting patient outcomes, guiding treatment decisions, and informing clinical management strategies in glioblastoma. By incorporating age, Karnofsky Performance Status, extent of surgical resection, molecular biomarkers, molecular subtypes, and treatment response into prognostic assessment, clinicians can tailor personalized therapeutic approaches to optimize patient outcomes and improve survival in this challenging disease. As the field of glioblastoma research continues to evolve, further elucidation of prognostic factors and their clinical implications will be essential for advancing precision medicine and optimizing patient care in glioblastoma management.

Harnessing Predictive Models and Scoring Systems in Glioblastoma: Enhancing Prognostic Accuracy and Clinical Decision-Making

Glioblastoma, characterized by its aggressive behavior and heterogeneous clinical course, presents significant challenges for prognostic assessment and treatment planning. Predictive models and scoring systems offer valuable tools for predicting patient outcomes, guiding therapeutic decisions, and optimizing clinical management strategies in glioblastoma. In this comprehensive exploration, we delve into the diverse array of predictive models and scoring systems utilized in glioblastoma, unraveling their significance, clinical applications, and potential for enhancing prognostic accuracy and personalized care.

1. Recursive Partitioning Analysis (RPA):

- **Development:** Recursive partitioning analysis (RPA) is a statistical method used to stratify patients into prognostic groups based on key clinical and demographic factors, such as age, Karnofsky Performance Status (KPS), and extent of surgical resection.
- **Clinical Utility:** RPA-derived prognostic scores provide valuable prognostic information and guide treatment decisions in glioblastoma, enabling risk stratification, prognostic assessment, and therapeutic planning

based on individual patient characteristics and disease status.

2. Glioma Grading Systems:

- **WHO Classification and Grading:** The World Health Organization (WHO) classification system for gliomas stratifies tumors into grades I-IV based on histological features, molecular alterations, and clinical behavior, with higher grades associated with greater aggressiveness and poorer prognosis.
- **Clinical Applications:** Glioma grading systems inform treatment decisions, prognostic assessment, and clinical trial eligibility in glioblastoma patients, facilitating personalized therapeutic approaches tailored to the tumor's grade, molecular subtype, and prognostic profile.

3. Molecular Profiling and Genomic Signatures:

- **MGMT Promoter Methylation Status:** Methylation of the O6-methylguanine-DNA methyltransferase (MGMT) promoter is predictive of response to alkylating chemotherapy agents, such as temozolomide, and is associated with improved prognosis and longer survival in glioblastoma patients.
- **IDH Mutation Status:** Mutations in the isocitrate dehydrogenase (IDH) genes, particularly IDH1 R132H, are associated with distinct clinical characteristics, improved prognosis, and better response to therapy in glioblastoma patients, guiding treatment selection and prognostic assessment.

4. Nomograms and Prognostic Scores:

- **Development:** Nomograms and prognostic scores integrate multiple clinical, pathological, and molecular factors into a comprehensive predictive model, enabling personalized prognostic assessment and

treatment planning in glioblastoma patients.
- **Clinical Applications:** Nomograms and prognostic scores provide individualized estimates of survival, recurrence risk, and treatment response in glioblastoma patients, facilitating shared decision-making, patient counseling, and therapeutic optimization based on personalized risk profiles.

5. **Radiomics and Imaging Biomarkers:**
   - **Radiomic Features:** Radiomics utilizes advanced image analysis techniques to extract quantitative features from medical imaging data, such as magnetic resonance imaging (MRI) and computed tomography (CT), enabling non-invasive assessment of tumor characteristics, heterogeneity, and treatment response.
   - **Predictive Models:** Radiomic-based predictive models and imaging biomarkers offer valuable insights into tumor biology, treatment response, and prognosis in glioblastoma, guiding treatment planning, response assessment, and surveillance strategies based on imaging-based risk stratification.

6. **Machine Learning and Artificial Intelligence (AI):**
   - **Algorithm Development:** Machine learning and artificial intelligence (AI) algorithms leverage computational methods to analyze large datasets, identify patterns, and develop predictive models for prognostic assessment, treatment response prediction, and therapeutic decision-making in glioblastoma.
   - **Clinical Integration:** Machine learning-based predictive models and AI algorithms hold promise for enhancing prognostic accuracy, optimizing treatment strategies, and personalizing care in glioblastoma management, facilitating real-time decision support and precision medicine approaches tailored to

individual patient characteristics and tumor biology.

Conclusion: Predictive models and scoring systems play a crucial role in prognostic assessment, treatment planning, and clinical management strategies in glioblastoma. By integrating clinical, pathological, molecular, and imaging data into comprehensive predictive models, clinicians can optimize patient outcomes, improve survival, and enhance personalized care in this challenging disease. As the field of predictive modeling and precision medicine continues to evolve, further refinement and validation of predictive models and scoring systems will be essential for advancing prognostic accuracy and optimizing therapeutic approaches in glioblastoma management.

Unraveling the Significance of Biomarkers in Prognostic Assessment of Glioblastoma: A Roadmap to Personalized Care

Glioblastoma, with its aggressive behavior and variable clinical outcomes, necessitates accurate prognostic assessment to guide treatment decisions and optimize patient care. Biomarkers, encompassing a diverse array of molecular, genetic, and imaging markers, offer valuable insights into tumor biology, treatment response, and prognosis in glioblastoma. In this comprehensive exploration, we delve into the pivotal role of biomarkers in prognostic assessment, unraveling their significance, clinical implications, and potential for guiding personalized therapeutic approaches in glioblastoma management.

1. Genetic Biomarkers:

- **IDH Mutation Status:** Mutations in the isocitrate dehydrogenase (IDH) genes, particularly IDH1 R132H, are associated with improved prognosis, longer survival, and distinct clinical characteristics in glioblastoma patients, guiding treatment selection and prognostic assessment.

- **MGMT Promoter Methylation:** Methylation of the O6-methylguanine-DNA methyltransferase (MGMT) promoter is predictive of response to alkylating chemotherapy agents, such as temozolomide, and is associated with improved prognosis and longer survival in glioblastoma patients.

2. **Molecular Biomarkers:**
   - **EGFR Amplification:** Amplification of the epidermal growth factor receptor (EGFR) gene is a common molecular alteration in glioblastoma, associated with tumor aggressiveness, treatment resistance, and poorer prognosis, highlighting the importance of EGFR as a prognostic biomarker.
   - **TERT Promoter Mutations:** Mutations in the telomerase reverse transcriptase (TERT) promoter are associated with aggressive clinical behavior, shorter survival, and poorer prognosis in glioblastoma patients, serving as a prognostic biomarker for risk stratification and prognostic assessment.

3. **Imaging Biomarkers:**
   - **Radiomic Features:** Radiomics utilizes advanced image analysis techniques to extract quantitative features from medical imaging data, such as magnetic resonance imaging (MRI) and computed tomography (CT), enabling non-invasive assessment of tumor characteristics, heterogeneity, and treatment response.
   - **Perfusion Imaging:** Perfusion imaging techniques, such as dynamic contrast-enhanced MRI (DCE-MRI) and perfusion-weighted imaging (PWI), provide valuable insights into tumor vascularity, microvascular density, and blood-brain barrier permeability, serving as imaging biomarkers for prognostic assessment and treatment response

prediction.

4. Immune Biomarkers:

- **Tumor-Infiltrating Lymphocytes (TILs):** The presence of tumor-infiltrating lymphocytes (TILs) within the tumor microenvironment is associated with improved prognosis, longer survival, and better treatment response in glioblastoma patients, reflecting enhanced antitumor immunity and immune surveillance.
- **PD-L1 Expression:** Expression of programmed death-ligand 1 (PD-L1) in glioblastoma tumors is associated with immune evasion, tumor immune escape, and treatment resistance, serving as a potential biomarker for immunotherapy response prediction and prognostic assessment.

5. Circulating Biomarkers:

- **Circulating Tumor DNA (ctDNA):** Circulating tumor DNA (ctDNA), released into the bloodstream from tumor cells, serves as a non-invasive biomarker for monitoring tumor dynamics, treatment response, and disease progression in glioblastoma patients, facilitating real-time prognostic assessment and treatment monitoring.

6. Integration of Biomarkers:

- **Multimodal Approach:** Integrating multiple biomarkers, including genetic, molecular, imaging, and immune markers, into a multimodal prognostic model enhances prognostic accuracy, improves risk stratification, and guides personalized therapeutic approaches in glioblastoma management.
- **Precision Medicine:** Biomarker-driven precision medicine approaches, tailored to individual patient characteristics and tumor biology, optimize treatment selection, improve patient outcomes, and enhance

survival in glioblastoma patients, paving the way for personalized care in this devastating disease.

Conclusion: Biomarkers play a pivotal role in prognostic assessment, treatment planning, and personalized care in glioblastoma. By unraveling the complex interplay of genetic, molecular, imaging, and immune markers, clinicians can optimize prognostic accuracy, guide therapeutic decisions, and improve patient outcomes in this challenging disease. As the field of biomarker research continues to evolve, further elucidation and validation of biomarkers will be essential for advancing prognostic assessment, optimizing treatment strategies, and enhancing personalized care in glioblastoma management.

CHAPTER 7: TREATMENT APPROACHES

Navigating Glioblastoma Surgery: Principles, Techniques, and Advances

Surgery serves as a cornerstone in the multimodal management of glioblastoma, offering the potential for tumor debulking, symptom relief, and histopathological diagnosis. The principles and techniques of glioblastoma surgery have evolved significantly over the years, driven by advances in neuroimaging, surgical navigation, intraoperative monitoring, and minimally invasive approaches. In this comprehensive exploration, we delve into the intricacies of glioblastoma surgery, unraveling its principles, techniques, and recent advances that have transformed surgical management and improved patient outcomes.

1. Preoperative Considerations:

- **Neuroimaging:** High-resolution magnetic resonance imaging (MRI), including contrast-enhanced sequences and functional imaging modalities, such as diffusion tensor imaging (DTI) and functional MRI (fMRI), plays a crucial role in preoperative planning, tumor localization, and identification of eloquent brain regions.
- **Surgical Navigation:** Advanced surgical navigation systems, incorporating intraoperative MRI,

neuronavigation, and stereotactic guidance, facilitate precise localization of tumor margins, optimal trajectory planning, and real-time intraoperative navigation to enhance surgical accuracy and minimize collateral damage to adjacent brain structures.

2. Surgical Approaches:

- **Craniotomy:** Open craniotomy remains the standard surgical approach for glioblastoma resection, providing direct access to the tumor, maximal tumor debulking, and histopathological diagnosis.
- **Minimally Invasive Techniques:** Minimally invasive approaches, including keyhole craniotomy, endoscopic-assisted surgery, and laser interstitial thermal therapy (LITT), offer alternatives to traditional craniotomy, enabling targeted tumor ablation, minimal brain manipulation, and shorter hospital stays with reduced morbidity.

3. Intraoperative Monitoring:

- **Electrophysiological Monitoring:** Intraoperative electrophysiological monitoring, including motor and sensory evoked potentials (MEPs and SSEPs) and electrocorticography (ECoG), enables real-time assessment of neurological function and identification of eloquent brain areas to minimize the risk of postoperative deficits.
- **Awake Surgery:** Awake craniotomy with intraoperative brain mapping allows for functional mapping of eloquent brain regions, such as language and motor areas, facilitating maximal tumor resection while preserving essential neurological function.

4. Surgical Resection:

- **Maximal Safe Resection:** The goal of glioblastoma surgery is maximal safe resection, aiming to achieve the maximal extent of tumor removal

while preserving critical neurological function and minimizing the risk of surgical morbidity.
- **Subtotal Resection:** In cases where complete resection is not feasible due to tumor location or proximity to eloquent brain regions, subtotal resection or debulking may be performed to alleviate mass effect, relieve symptoms, and facilitate adjuvant therapies.

5. **Tumor Resection Techniques:**
   - **Cavitron Ultrasonic Aspiration (CUSA):** Ultrasonic aspirators, such as the Cavitron Ultrasonic Surgical Aspirator (CUSA), facilitate gentle tissue dissection and precise tumor debulking by breaking down tumor tissue while preserving adjacent normal brain parenchyma.
   - **Neuro-Navigation:** Intraoperative neuronavigation systems provide real-time guidance for tumor localization, trajectory planning, and surgical resection, enhancing surgical accuracy and facilitating targeted tumor removal.

6. **Postoperative Care and Management:**
   - **Neurocritical Care:** Postoperative neurocritical care, including close monitoring of neurological status, management of intracranial pressure (ICP), and prevention of complications, such as cerebral edema and surgical site infections, is essential for optimizing patient outcomes and facilitating early recovery.
   - **Adjuvant Therapies:** Adjuvant therapies, including radiation therapy and chemotherapy, are typically initiated following surgical resection to target residual tumor cells, delay tumor recurrence, and improve long-term survival in glioblastoma patients.

7. **Recent Advances and Innovations:**
   - **Intraoperative Imaging:** Intraoperative imaging modalities, such as intraoperative MRI

and intraoperative ultrasound, enable real-time visualization of tumor margins, assessment of extent of resection, and immediate feedback to guide surgical decision-making and optimize tumor removal.

- **Fluorescence-Guided Surgery:** Fluorescence-guided surgery utilizing intraoperative fluorescent dyes, such as 5-aminolevulinic acid (5-ALA) and fluorescein, enhances tumor visualization, delineation of tumor margins, and extent of resection, improving surgical outcomes and patient survival.

Conclusion: Glioblastoma surgery represents a crucial component of multimodal treatment, offering the potential for tumor debulking, symptom relief, and histopathological diagnosis. By adhering to the principles of maximal safe resection, utilizing advanced surgical techniques and technologies, and incorporating recent advances and innovations, clinicians can optimize surgical outcomes, improve patient survival, and enhance quality of life in glioblastoma patients. As the field continues to evolve, further refinement of surgical approaches and integration of novel technologies will be essential for advancing surgical management and optimizing patient care in this devastating disease.

Illuminating Glioblastoma Treatment: A Radiant Perspective on Radiation Therapy

Radiation therapy stands as a cornerstone in the multimodal management of glioblastoma, offering the potential to target residual tumor cells, delay tumor progression, and improve patient outcomes. Over the years, both conventional and advanced radiation techniques have evolved, driven by technological advancements and a deeper understanding of tumor biology. In this comprehensive exploration, we delve into the principles, techniques, and recent advances in radiation therapy for glioblastoma, illuminating the path towards optimized treatment strategies and enhanced patient care.

1. **Principles of Radiation Therapy:**
   - **Radiation Sensitivity:** Glioblastoma cells exhibit varying degrees of sensitivity to ionizing radiation, with high proliferative rates and genetic heterogeneity contributing to differential responses to radiation therapy.
   - **Fractionation:** Fractionated radiation therapy delivers the total prescribed dose of radiation in multiple smaller fractions over several weeks, allowing for tumor cell repopulation and normal tissue repair between treatment sessions while minimizing the risk of radiation-induced toxicity.

2. **Conventional Radiation Techniques:**
   - **External Beam Radiation Therapy (EBRT):** EBRT remains the standard approach for delivering radiation therapy to glioblastoma patients, utilizing high-energy X-rays or protons to target the tumor while sparing surrounding normal brain tissue.
   - **Three-Dimensional Conformal Radiation Therapy (3DCRT):** 3DCRT utilizes computerized treatment planning to deliver radiation beams from multiple angles, conforming to the shape and size of the tumor while minimizing exposure to adjacent critical structures.

3. **Advanced Radiation Techniques:**
   - **Intensity-Modulated Radiation Therapy (IMRT):** IMRT delivers highly conformal radiation doses by modulating the intensity of radiation beams, allowing for precise targeting of the tumor while sparing nearby organs at risk, such as the optic nerves and brainstem.
   - **Stereotactic Radiosurgery (SRS):** SRS delivers a high dose of radiation to the tumor with submillimeter

accuracy, utilizing precise targeting and multiple radiation beams to deliver a focused dose while minimizing exposure to surrounding healthy tissue.

4. Novel Approaches in Radiation Therapy:

- **Proton Beam Therapy:** Proton beam therapy offers the potential for improved dose distribution and reduced radiation exposure to normal brain tissue compared to conventional photon-based radiation therapy, minimizing the risk of radiation-induced toxicity and long-term side effects.
- **Particle Therapy:** Particle therapy, including carbon ion therapy and heavy ion therapy, delivers high-linear energy transfer (LET) radiation to the tumor, resulting in enhanced tumor cell killing and potential synergistic effects with conventional radiation therapy.

5. Radiosensitizers and Targeted Therapies:

- **Temozolomide (TMZ):** Concurrent and adjuvant temozolomide chemotherapy, in combination with radiation therapy, has become standard of care for glioblastoma patients, enhancing radiation sensitivity and improving overall survival.
- **Targeted Therapies:** Targeted agents, such as anti-angiogenic agents (e.g., bevacizumab) and molecularly targeted inhibitors (e.g., EGFR inhibitors), may enhance the efficacy of radiation therapy by targeting specific molecular pathways involved in tumor growth and progression.

6. Adverse Effects and Management:

- **Acute Toxicity:** Acute radiation-induced toxicity, including fatigue, nausea, and headaches, is common during and immediately following radiation therapy and is managed symptomatically with supportive care and medications.

- **Late Toxicity:** Late radiation-induced toxicity, such as radiation necrosis, cognitive decline, and radiation-induced secondary malignancies, may occur months to years after treatment completion and require long-term monitoring and management.

7. **Future Directions and Emerging Technologies:**
    - **Immunotherapy and Radiobiology:** Combining radiation therapy with immunotherapy holds promise for enhancing antitumor immune responses, overcoming immune evasion mechanisms, and improving treatment outcomes in glioblastoma patients.
    - **Radiomics and Artificial Intelligence:** Radiomics-based predictive models and artificial intelligence algorithms enable personalized treatment planning, response prediction, and outcome assessment in glioblastoma patients, facilitating precision medicine approaches tailored to individual patient characteristics and tumor biology.

Conclusion: Radiation therapy plays a pivotal role in the multimodal management of glioblastoma, offering the potential to target residual tumor cells, delay tumor progression, and improve patient outcomes. By harnessing both conventional and advanced radiation techniques, integrating novel approaches and targeted therapies, and embracing emerging technologies, clinicians can optimize radiation therapy delivery, minimize treatment-related toxicity, and enhance overall survival in glioblastoma patients. As the field continues to evolve, further refinements in radiation techniques, personalized treatment approaches, and interdisciplinary collaborations will be essential for advancing radiation therapy and improving patient care in this challenging disease.

Exploring Chemotherapy in Glioblastoma: Current Agents and

Novel Frontiers

Chemotherapy plays a pivotal role in the multimodal treatment of glioblastoma, offering the potential to target proliferating tumor cells, inhibit angiogenesis, and enhance radiosensitivity. Over the years, numerous chemotherapeutic agents have been investigated, both as single agents and in combination regimens, aiming to improve patient outcomes and overcome treatment resistance. In this comprehensive exploration, we delve into the current landscape of chemotherapy for glioblastoma, examining existing agents, novel approaches, and emerging frontiers that hold promise for advancing treatment efficacy and patient survival.

1. Current Chemotherapeutic Agents:

- **Temozolomide (TMZ):** TMZ, an oral alkylating agent, represents the standard chemotherapy for glioblastoma, administered concurrently with radiation therapy followed by adjuvant maintenance therapy. Its mechanism of action involves DNA methylation, leading to tumor cell death and apoptosis.
- **Carmustine (BCNU):** Carmustine, a nitrosourea alkylating agent, has demonstrated efficacy in glioblastoma as both a single agent and in combination regimens. It exerts its antitumor effects by alkylating DNA, inhibiting DNA replication, and inducing cytotoxicity.
- **Lomustine (CCNU):** Lomustine, another nitrosourea alkylating agent, is commonly used in the treatment of recurrent glioblastoma, either as monotherapy or in combination with other chemotherapeutic agents. Its mechanism of action involves DNA alkylation and interference with DNA synthesis and repair mechanisms.

2. Novel Approaches in Chemotherapy:

- **Targeted Therapies:** Targeted agents, such as anti-angiogenic agents (e.g., bevacizumab), epidermal growth factor receptor (EGFR) inhibitors (e.g., erlotinib), and mammalian target of rapamycin (mTOR) inhibitors (e.g., temsirolimus), have been investigated for their potential to inhibit specific molecular pathways implicated in glioblastoma growth and progression.
- **Immunotherapy:** Immunotherapy approaches, including immune checkpoint inhibitors (e.g., pembrolizumab), chimeric antigen receptor (CAR) T-cell therapy, and cancer vaccines, aim to harness the immune system to target glioblastoma cells, overcome immune evasion mechanisms, and induce antitumor immune responses.
- **Nanotechnology:** Nanoparticle-based drug delivery systems, such as liposomes, polymeric nanoparticles, and dendrimers, offer the potential for targeted drug delivery, enhanced drug penetration across the blood-brain barrier, and reduced systemic toxicity in glioblastoma patients.

3. **Combination Chemotherapy Regimens:**
   - **Stupp Protocol:** The Stupp protocol, consisting of concurrent TMZ and radiation therapy followed by adjuvant TMZ maintenance therapy, remains the standard of care for newly diagnosed glioblastoma patients, demonstrating improved overall survival compared to radiation therapy alone.
   - **Multimodal Regimens:** Multimodal chemotherapy regimens, incorporating multiple chemotherapeutic agents, targeted therapies, and immunotherapy approaches, are being investigated in clinical trials to optimize treatment efficacy, overcome treatment resistance, and improve patient outcomes in

glioblastoma.

4. Resistance Mechanisms and Overcoming Resistance:

- **O6-Methylguanine-DNA Methyltransferase (MGMT) Expression:** Expression of MGMT, a DNA repair enzyme, confers resistance to alkylating agents, such as TMZ, by repairing DNA damage induced by chemotherapy. Strategies to overcome MGMT-mediated resistance include MGMT promoter methylation and combination therapy with MGMT inhibitors.

- **Tumor Microenvironment:** The tumor microenvironment, characterized by hypoxia, immune suppression, and aberrant angiogenesis, plays a crucial role in mediating resistance to chemotherapy in glioblastoma. Targeting the tumor microenvironment with anti-angiogenic agents, immunotherapy approaches, and stromal-targeting agents may help overcome resistance and enhance treatment efficacy.

5. Personalized Medicine Approaches:

- **Molecular Profiling:** Molecular profiling of glioblastoma tumors enables identification of specific molecular alterations, such as IDH mutations, EGFR amplification, and PTEN loss, guiding treatment selection and personalized therapeutic approaches tailored to individual patient characteristics and tumor biology.

- **Biomarker-Guided Therapy:** Biomarker-driven treatment strategies, including MGMT promoter methylation status, molecular subtyping, and immune checkpoint expression, inform treatment decisions and predict response to chemotherapy, facilitating personalized medicine approaches in glioblastoma management.

6. Challenges and Future Directions:

- **Drug Delivery Challenges:** Overcoming the blood-brain barrier, achieving adequate drug penetration into the tumor, and minimizing systemic toxicity remain significant challenges in glioblastoma chemotherapy, necessitating innovative drug delivery strategies and nanotechnology-based approaches.
- **Drug Resistance Mechanisms:** Elucidating the molecular mechanisms underlying chemotherapy resistance, such as tumor heterogeneity, clonal evolution, and adaptive resistance, is essential for developing targeted therapies and combination regimens to overcome resistance and improve treatment outcomes in glioblastoma patients.

Conclusion: Chemotherapy plays a crucial role in the multimodal management of glioblastoma, offering the potential to target proliferating tumor cells, inhibit angiogenesis, and enhance radiosensitivity. By embracing both current agents and novel approaches, integrating targeted therapies and immunotherapy, and advancing personalized medicine approaches, clinicians can optimize treatment efficacy, overcome treatment resistance, and improve patient outcomes in this challenging disease. As the field continues to evolve, further refinements in chemotherapy strategies, drug delivery technologies, and biomarker-guided therapies will be essential for advancing glioblastoma treatment and enhancing patient care.

Advancing Precision Medicine: Targeted Therapies in Glioblastoma

Targeted therapies represent a promising frontier in the management of glioblastoma, offering the potential to selectively inhibit specific molecular pathways implicated in tumor growth and progression. Among these targeted approaches, inhibitors of epidermal growth factor receptor

(EGFR), angiogenesis, and other key signaling pathways have garnered significant interest for their potential to overcome treatment resistance and improve patient outcomes. In this exploration, we delve into the landscape of targeted therapies in glioblastoma, focusing on EGFR inhibitors, angiogenesis inhibitors, and emerging approaches that hold promise for advancing precision medicine in this challenging disease.

1. EGFR Inhibitors:

- **Erlotinib (Tarceva):** Erlotinib is an oral EGFR tyrosine kinase inhibitor (TKI) that blocks the activation of EGFR signaling pathways implicated in glioblastoma growth and progression. Clinical trials evaluating erlotinib in glioblastoma have shown limited efficacy as monotherapy but have demonstrated potential synergistic effects in combination with other targeted agents or chemotherapy.
- **Gefitinib (Iressa):** Gefitinib, another EGFR TKI, has been investigated in clinical trials for its potential to inhibit EGFR signaling and overcome EGFR-mediated resistance in glioblastoma. While initial studies showed modest activity, subsequent trials have failed to demonstrate significant clinical benefit as monotherapy or in combination regimens.

2. Angiogenesis Inhibitors:

- **Bevacizumab (Avastin):** Bevacizumab is a monoclonal antibody targeting vascular endothelial growth factor (VEGF), a key mediator of angiogenesis and tumor neovascularization in glioblastoma. It has been approved for the treatment of recurrent glioblastoma based on clinical trials demonstrating improvement in progression-free survival and radiographic response rates, although overall survival benefits remain modest.
- **Aflibercept (Zaltrap):** Aflibercept is a soluble decoy

receptor that binds to VEGF-A, VEGF-B, and placental growth factor (PlGF), thereby inhibiting angiogenesis and tumor vascularization. Clinical trials evaluating aflibercept in glioblastoma have shown mixed results, with some studies demonstrating modest efficacy in recurrent disease settings.

3. Other Targeted Therapies:

- **mTOR Inhibitors:** Mammalian target of rapamycin (mTOR) inhibitors, such as temsirolimus and everolimus, target the mTOR signaling pathway, which regulates cell growth, proliferation, and survival. Clinical trials investigating mTOR inhibitors in glioblastoma have shown variable responses, with limited efficacy as monotherapy but potential synergistic effects in combination regimens.
- **PARP Inhibitors:** Poly(ADP-ribose) polymerase (PARP) inhibitors, such as olaparib and veliparib, target the DNA repair pathway and have shown preclinical activity in glioblastoma models, particularly in tumors with homologous recombination deficiency (HRD) or mutations in DNA repair genes.

4. Challenges and Future Directions:

- **Resistance Mechanisms:** Tumor heterogeneity, adaptive resistance mechanisms, and compensatory signaling pathways pose significant challenges to the effectiveness of targeted therapies in glioblastoma, necessitating combination approaches, rational drug selection, and biomarker-guided strategies to overcome resistance and improve treatment outcomes.
- **Blood-Brain Barrier (BBB) Penetration:** Limited penetration of targeted agents across the blood-brain barrier (BBB) remains a major hurdle in glioblastoma therapy, highlighting the need for innovative drug

delivery approaches, such as nanoparticle-based formulations and focused ultrasound-mediated BBB disruption, to enhance drug delivery to the central nervous system.

5. **Emerging Strategies and Personalized Medicine:**
   - **Immunotherapy Combinations:** Combining targeted therapies with immunotherapy approaches, such as immune checkpoint inhibitors and chimeric antigen receptor (CAR) T-cell therapy, holds promise for enhancing antitumor immune responses, overcoming immune evasion mechanisms, and improving treatment outcomes in glioblastoma patients.
   - **Biomarker-Guided Therapy:** Biomarker-driven treatment strategies, including molecular profiling, EGFR mutation status, and angiogenesis biomarkers, inform treatment decisions and predict response to targeted therapies, facilitating personalized medicine approaches tailored to individual patient characteristics and tumor biology.

Conclusion: Targeted therapies represent a promising avenue for advancing precision medicine in glioblastoma, offering the potential to selectively inhibit specific molecular pathways implicated in tumor growth and progression. By embracing EGFR inhibitors, angiogenesis inhibitors, and emerging approaches, clinicians can optimize treatment efficacy, overcome treatment resistance, and improve patient outcomes in this challenging disease. As the field continues to evolve, further refinements in targeted therapy strategies, combination approaches, and personalized medicine approaches will be essential for advancing precision medicine and enhancing patient care in glioblastoma management.

Revolutionizing Glioblastoma Treatment: Immunotherapy at the Forefront

Immunotherapy has emerged as a promising frontier in the management of glioblastoma, harnessing the power of the immune system to target and eliminate tumor cells. Among the diverse array of immunotherapy approaches, checkpoint inhibitors, cancer vaccines, and chimeric antigen receptor (CAR) T-cell therapy have garnered significant attention for their potential to overcome immune evasion mechanisms and induce durable antitumor immune responses. In this comprehensive exploration, we delve into the landscape of immunotherapy in glioblastoma, examining the mechanisms of action, clinical efficacy, and future directions of checkpoint inhibitors, vaccines, and CAR-T cell therapy in reshaping the treatment paradigm of this devastating disease.

1. **Checkpoint Inhibitors:**
   - **Programmed Death-1 (PD-1) Inhibitors:** PD-1 inhibitors, such as pembrolizumab and nivolumab, target the PD-1 receptor on T cells, blocking the interaction with its ligands (PD-L1/PD-L2) expressed on tumor cells and inhibiting immune checkpoint signaling pathways. Clinical trials evaluating PD-1 inhibitors in glioblastoma have shown modest efficacy, with durable responses observed in a subset of patients.
   - **Cytotoxic T-Lymphocyte-Associated Protein 4 (CTLA-4) Inhibitors:** CTLA-4 inhibitors, such as ipilimumab, target the CTLA-4 receptor on T cells, enhancing T cell activation and proliferation while attenuating immune suppression. Combination strategies with PD-1 inhibitors or other immunotherapeutic agents are being investigated to enhance antitumor immune responses and overcome resistance mechanisms in glioblastoma.

2. **Cancer Vaccines:**
   - **Peptide Vaccines:** Peptide vaccines, consisting of

tumor-associated antigens (TAAs) or neoantigens derived from glioblastoma cells, stimulate the immune system to recognize and target tumor-specific antigens, eliciting an antitumor immune response. Clinical trials evaluating peptide vaccines, such as the EGFRvIII peptide vaccine (rindopepimut), have shown promising results in select patient populations, with improved progression-free survival and immune responses observed.

- **Dendritic Cell Vaccines:** Dendritic cell vaccines, generated from patients' own dendritic cells pulsed with tumor antigens, are designed to activate and enhance antigen-specific T cell responses against glioblastoma cells. Early-phase clinical trials investigating dendritic cell vaccines have demonstrated safety, immunogenicity, and potential clinical benefit in glioblastoma patients, warranting further evaluation in larger cohorts.

3. CAR-T Cell Therapy:

- **Tumor-Specific CAR-T Cells:** CAR-T cell therapy involves genetically engineering patients' T cells to express chimeric antigen receptors (CARs) targeting tumor-specific antigens, such as EGFRvIII or IL-13Rα2, expressed on glioblastoma cells. Phase I/II clinical trials evaluating CAR-T cell therapy in glioblastoma have shown feasibility, safety, and preliminary efficacy, with durable responses observed in some patients.
- **Bispecific CAR-T Cells:** Bispecific CAR-T cells, engineered to recognize multiple tumor antigens or engage additional immune effector cells, offer the potential for enhanced tumor targeting, improved specificity, and augmented antitumor immune responses in glioblastoma patients.

4. Challenges and Future Directions:

- **Tumor Microenvironment:** The immunosuppressive tumor microenvironment, characterized by regulatory T cells, myeloid-derived suppressor cells (MDSCs), and inhibitory cytokines, poses significant challenges to the effectiveness of immunotherapy in glioblastoma, highlighting the need for combination strategies targeting multiple immune checkpoints and modulating the tumor microenvironment.
- **Patient Selection and Biomarkers:** Biomarker-driven patient selection and monitoring are critical for identifying responders, predicting treatment outcomes, and optimizing immunotherapy approaches in glioblastoma. Biomarkers, such as PD-L1 expression, tumor mutational burden (TMB), and immune cell infiltrates, may inform treatment decisions and guide personalized immunotherapy strategies tailored to individual patient characteristics and tumor biology.

5. Combination Strategies and Personalized Medicine:
- **Combination Therapy:** Combining immunotherapy with standard-of-care treatments, such as radiation therapy, chemotherapy, and targeted therapies, offers the potential for synergistic effects, enhanced treatment efficacy, and improved patient outcomes in glioblastoma. Rational combination strategies targeting complementary pathways and overcoming resistance mechanisms are being investigated in clinical trials to optimize immunotherapy approaches.
- **Personalized Medicine:** Personalized medicine approaches, integrating molecular profiling, immune profiling, and biomarker-guided therapy selection, enable tailored immunotherapy strategies based on individual patient characteristics and tumor biology, maximizing treatment efficacy and

minimizing treatment-related toxicity in glioblastoma management.

Conclusion: Immunotherapy holds tremendous promise for transforming the treatment landscape of glioblastoma, offering the potential to harness the immune system to target and eliminate tumor cells. By embracing checkpoint inhibitors, cancer vaccines, CAR-T cell therapy, and combination strategies, clinicians can optimize treatment efficacy, overcome treatment resistance, and improve patient outcomes in this challenging disease. As the field continues to evolve, further refinements in immunotherapy approaches, patient selection strategies, and personalized medicine approaches will be essential for advancing immunotherapy and reshaping the treatment paradigm of glioblastoma.

Optimizing Care: Multimodal Approaches and Treatment Algorithms in Glioblastoma

Glioblastoma, a complex and aggressive brain tumor, poses significant challenges to treatment due to its infiltrative nature and resistance to standard therapies. To address these challenges, clinicians have increasingly embraced multimodal approaches that combine surgery, radiation therapy, chemotherapy, and emerging treatment modalities to improve outcomes for patients. In this comprehensive exploration, we delve into the rationale, principles, and evolving treatment algorithms guiding multimodal approaches in glioblastoma management, aiming to optimize care and enhance patient outcomes in this challenging disease.

1. Rationale for Multimodal Approaches:

- **Tumor Heterogeneity:** Glioblastoma exhibits significant intratumoral heterogeneity, with diverse molecular subtypes and cellular populations contributing to tumor growth, invasion, and treatment resistance. Multimodal approaches target different aspects of tumor biology, including tumor bulk, infiltrative cells, and resistant clones, to maximize treatment efficacy and overcome tumor heterogeneity.

- **Synergistic Effects:** Combining surgery, radiation therapy, and chemotherapy harnesses synergistic effects, targeting residual tumor cells, disrupting tumor microenvironment, and enhancing treatment response rates. Multimodal approaches aim to exploit complementary mechanisms of action and overcome resistance mechanisms to improve patient outcomes in glioblastoma.

2. Principles of Multimodal Treatment:

- **Maximal Safe Resection:** Surgery remains the cornerstone of multimodal treatment, aiming for maximal safe resection to debulk the tumor, relieve mass effect, and obtain tissue for histopathological diagnosis. Advanced surgical techniques, such as awake mapping and fluorescence-guided surgery, facilitate precise tumor removal while preserving critical neurological function.
- **Adjuvant Therapy:** Adjuvant therapies, including radiation therapy and chemotherapy, are initiated following surgery to target residual tumor cells and delay tumor progression. The Stupp protocol, consisting of concurrent temozolomide and radiation therapy followed by adjuvant temozolomide, represents the standard of care for newly diagnosed glioblastoma patients, improving overall survival and delaying disease progression.
- **Emerging Modalities:** Emerging treatment modalities, such as immunotherapy, targeted therapy, and tumor-treating fields (TTFields), are increasingly integrated into multimodal treatment algorithms to enhance treatment efficacy, overcome treatment resistance,

and improve patient outcomes in glioblastoma.

3. Treatment Algorithms:

- **Newly Diagnosed Glioblastoma:** For newly diagnosed glioblastoma, the treatment algorithm typically involves maximal safe resection followed by adjuvant chemoradiation with temozolomide. Emerging approaches, such as tumor-treating fields (TTFields) or immunotherapy combinations, may be considered in select patients to further optimize treatment outcomes.

- **Recurrent Glioblastoma:** In recurrent glioblastoma, treatment algorithms are less standardized and often tailored to individual patient characteristics, including performance status, extent of recurrence, and previous treatment history. Options may include repeat surgery, re-irradiation, salvage chemotherapy, targeted therapy, or enrollment in clinical trials investigating novel treatment approaches.

4. Personalized Medicine Approaches:

- **Molecular Profiling:** Molecular profiling of glioblastoma tumors enables personalized treatment selection based on specific molecular alterations, such as IDH mutations, MGMT promoter methylation status, and EGFR amplification. Biomarker-driven therapy selection guides treatment decisions and optimizes treatment efficacy in glioblastoma management.

- **Immune Profiling:** Immune profiling of glioblastoma tumors and the tumor microenvironment informs treatment strategies and predicts response to immunotherapy approaches, such as checkpoint inhibitors or CAR-T cell therapy. Immune biomarkers, such as PD-L1 expression or tumor-infiltrating lymphocytes, may guide patient selection and treatment response assessment in glioblastoma immunotherapy.

5. Challenges and Future Directions:

- **Treatment Resistance:** Treatment resistance remains a significant challenge in glioblastoma management, necessitating novel treatment approaches, combination strategies, and rational drug selection to overcome resistance mechanisms and improve treatment outcomes.

- **Interdisciplinary Collaboration:** Interdisciplinary collaboration between neurosurgeons, radiation oncologists, medical oncologists, and neuro-oncologists is essential for optimizing multimodal treatment approaches, integrating novel therapies, and coordinating care for glioblastoma patients across the treatment continuum.

Conclusion: Multimodal approaches play a pivotal role in the management of glioblastoma, combining surgery, radiation therapy, chemotherapy, and emerging treatment modalities to maximize treatment efficacy and improve patient outcomes. By adhering to the principles of multimodal treatment, embracing personalized medicine approaches, and fostering interdisciplinary collaboration, clinicians can optimize care and enhance survival in this challenging disease. As the field continues to evolve, further refinements in treatment algorithms, novel treatment modalities, and personalized medicine strategies will be essential for advancing glioblastoma management and improving patient outcomes.

Enhancing Quality of Life: Palliative Care and Symptom Management in Glioblastoma

Glioblastoma, a devastating brain tumor, presents a multitude of challenges to patients and their families, often accompanied by debilitating symptoms and complex psychosocial issues. Palliative care plays a crucial role in alleviating suffering, optimizing symptom management, and enhancing quality of life for patients living with glioblastoma. In this exploration, we delve into the principles, goals, and strategies of palliative care, highlighting the importance of a holistic approach to symptom management and supportive care in glioblastoma patients.

1. **Principles of Palliative Care:**
   - **Holistic Approach:** Palliative care adopts a holistic approach to care, addressing physical, psychological, social, and spiritual aspects of patient well-being. It focuses on alleviating suffering, improving quality of life, and supporting patients and their families throughout the illness trajectory.
   - **Early Integration:** Early integration of palliative care alongside curative treatments is recommended for patients with glioblastoma, allowing for proactive symptom management, psychosocial support, and advance care planning from the time of diagnosis through the end of life.

2. **Goals of Palliative Care:**
   - **Symptom Management:** Palliative care aims to optimize symptom management and relieve distressing symptoms commonly experienced by glioblastoma patients, including pain, nausea, fatigue, seizures, cognitive impairment, and psychological distress.
   - **Psychosocial Support:** Palliative care provides psychosocial support and counseling to patients and their families, addressing emotional, social, and spiritual needs, facilitating coping strategies, and enhancing quality of life throughout the illness journey.
   - **Advance Care Planning:** Palliative care encourages

advance care planning discussions, empowering patients to make informed decisions about their goals of care, treatment preferences, and end-of-life wishes, ensuring that care aligns with patients' values and preferences.

3. Symptom Management Strategies:

- **Pain Management:** Pain in glioblastoma patients may result from tumor-related compression, inflammation, or treatment-related side effects. Multimodal analgesic approaches, including pharmacological interventions, such as opioids, adjuvant medications, and interventional procedures, are employed to effectively manage pain while minimizing adverse effects.

- **Nausea and Vomiting:** Nausea and vomiting, common symptoms in glioblastoma patients, may arise from tumor location, increased intracranial pressure, or side effects of chemotherapy. Antiemetic medications, hydration, dietary modifications, and behavioral interventions are utilized to alleviate symptoms and improve quality of life.

- **Fatigue Management:** Fatigue is a pervasive symptom in glioblastoma patients, impacting physical function, cognitive abilities, and overall well-being. Energy conservation techniques, physical activity, psychosocial support, and pharmacological interventions may help manage fatigue and enhance functional capacity.

- **Seizure Control:** Seizures are a frequent complication of glioblastoma, affecting quality of life and functional independence. Antiepileptic medications, seizure precautions, lifestyle modifications, and neurosurgical interventions are employed to control seizures and minimize their impact on daily activities.

4. **Psychosocial Support and Coping Strategies:**
    - **Counseling and Psychotherapy:** Counseling and psychotherapy services, including individual counseling, family therapy, and support groups, provide emotional support, coping strategies, and a safe space for patients and their families to process their experiences, fears, and concerns.
    - **Mindfulness and Relaxation Techniques:** Mindfulness-based interventions, relaxation techniques, guided imagery, and meditation practices offer stress reduction, promote emotional well-being, and enhance coping skills in glioblastoma patients facing the challenges of their diagnosis and treatment.
    - **Spiritual Care:** Spiritual care, encompassing existential support, religious counseling, and existential exploration, addresses patients' spiritual needs, beliefs, and values, providing comfort, meaning, and a sense of connection during difficult times.

5. **End-of-Life Care and Bereavement Support:**
    - **Hospice Care:** Hospice care provides compassionate end-of-life care for patients with advanced glioblastoma, focusing on comfort, dignity, and quality of life in the final stages of the illness. Hospice services offer symptom management, psychosocial support, and bereavement care for patients and their families.
    - **Bereavement Support:** Bereavement support services offer ongoing support and counseling to families following the loss of a loved one to glioblastoma, facilitating coping with grief, adjustment to loss, and the transition to life after bereavement.

6. **Caregiver Support and Respite Care:**
    - **Caregiver Support:** Caregivers play a vital role in

the care of glioblastoma patients, providing physical, emotional, and practical support throughout the illness journey. Caregiver support services offer education, training, respite care, and emotional support to alleviate caregiver burden and promote well-being.

- **Respite Care:** Respite care services provide temporary relief for caregivers, allowing them to take breaks, attend to their own needs, and recharge while ensuring that patients receive high-quality care and support in their absence.

Conclusion: Palliative care plays an integral role in the comprehensive management of glioblastoma, offering symptom management, psychosocial support, and holistic care throughout the illness trajectory. By embracing a patient-centered approach, optimizing symptom management, and providing compassionate support to patients and their families, palliative care enhances quality of life, promotes dignity, and fosters a sense of comfort and well-being in the face of a challenging diagnosis. As an essential component of glioblastoma care, palliative care empowers patients to live fully and comfortably, ensuring that their physical, emotional, and spiritual needs are addressed with compassion and dignity.

CHAPTER 8: EMERGING THERAPIES AND FUTURE DIRECTIONS

Exploring Novel Molecular Targets and Pathways in Glioblastoma Research

Glioblastoma, characterized by its aggressive nature and resistance to conventional therapies, continues to pose a significant clinical challenge. The identification of novel molecular targets and pathways holds promise for advancing the understanding of glioblastoma pathogenesis, overcoming treatment resistance, and improving patient outcomes. In this exploration, we delve into the emerging landscape of novel molecular targets and pathways in glioblastoma research, highlighting key discoveries, therapeutic implications, and future directions in the quest to transform glioblastoma treatment.

1. Cancer Stem Cells:

- **Identification and Characterization:** Cancer stem cells (CSCs) represent a subpopulation of tumor cells with self-renewal capacity and tumorigenic potential, contributing to tumor initiation, progression, and treatment resistance in glioblastoma. Novel molecular targets and pathways associated with CSCs, including Notch signaling, Hedgehog pathway, and Wnt/βcatenin pathway, are being investigated for their potential as therapeutic targets in glioblastoma.

2. Tumor Microenvironment:

- **Immune Checkpoints:** Immune checkpoint molecules, such as programmed cell death protein 1 (PD-1), programmed death-ligand 1 (PD-L1), and cytotoxic T-lymphocyte-associated protein 4 (CTLA-4), play a critical role in immune evasion and tumor immune escape in glioblastoma. Targeting immune checkpoints and modulating the tumor microenvironment offer promising strategies to enhance antitumor immune responses and overcome immunosuppression in glioblastoma.

3. Epigenetic Alterations:

- **Histone Modifications:** Epigenetic alterations, including histone modifications (e.g., histone methylation, acetylation, and ubiquitination), regulate gene expression and chromatin structure in glioblastoma, influencing tumor growth, invasion, and treatment response. Targeting epigenetic regulators and chromatin-modifying enzymes represents a novel therapeutic approach to modulate gene expression and reprogram tumor cell fate in glioblastoma.

4. Metabolic Reprogramming:

- **Glucose Metabolism:** Metabolic reprogramming is a hallmark of cancer, including glioblastoma, characterized by increased aerobic glycolysis (the Warburg effect) and altered metabolic pathways to support tumor growth and survival. Novel molecular targets and pathways involved in glucose metabolism, such as hexokinase 2 (HK2), pyruvate kinase M2 (PKM2), and lactate dehydrogenase A (LDHA), are under investigation for their potential as therapeutic targets in glioblastoma.

5. RNA Processing and Splicing:

- **Alternative Splicing:** Dysregulation of RNA processing and alternative splicing contributes to glioblastoma pathogenesis, generating tumor-specific isoforms and promoting tumor growth and invasion. Novel molecular targets and pathways involved in RNA processing and splicing, including spliceosome components, RNA-binding proteins, and splicing factors, are emerging as potential therapeutic targets in glioblastoma.

6. DNA Damage Response and Repair:

- **DNA Repair Pathways:** Glioblastoma cells exhibit dysregulated DNA damage response and repair mechanisms, leading to genomic instability and treatment resistance. Novel molecular targets and pathways associated with DNA repair pathways, such as poly(ADP-ribose) polymerase (PARP), ataxia telangiectasia mutated (ATM), and checkpoint kinase 1 (CHK1), are being explored for their potential as therapeutic targets in glioblastoma.

7. Extracellular Matrix Remodeling:

- **Matrix Metalloproteinases (MMPs):** Extracellular matrix (ECM) remodeling mediated by matrix metalloproteinases (MMPs) plays a critical role in glioblastoma invasion, angiogenesis, and metastasis. Novel molecular targets and pathways involved in ECM remodeling, such as MMP inhibitors, tissue inhibitors of metalloproteinases (TIMPs), and integrins, are under investigation for their potential as therapeutic targets in glioblastoma.

8. Challenges and Future Directions:

- **Drug Delivery and Penetration:** Overcoming the blood-brain barrier (BBB) and achieving adequate drug delivery and penetration into the central nervous system (CNS) remain significant challenges in glioblastoma treatment, necessitating innovative drug delivery strategies, nanoparticle-based formulations, and targeted delivery approaches to enhance therapeutic efficacy and minimize off-target effects.

- **Biomarker Identification:** Biomarker discovery and validation are essential for patient stratification, treatment selection, and response prediction in glioblastoma therapy. Identification of predictive biomarkers, such as molecular subtypes, genetic alterations, and treatment response markers, will facilitate personalized medicine approaches and improve patient outcomes in glioblastoma management.

Conclusion: The identification of novel molecular targets and pathways in glioblastoma research holds promise for advancing the understanding of tumor biology, overcoming treatment resistance, and improving patient outcomes. By exploring cancer stem cells, tumor microenvironment, epigenetic alterations, metabolic reprogramming, RNA processing, DNA damage response, and extracellular matrix remodeling, researchers aim to uncover new therapeutic vulnerabilities and develop targeted therapies tailored to the unique molecular characteristics of glioblastoma tumors. As the field continues to evolve, further elucidation of novel molecular targets and pathways will pave the way for innovative treatment strategies and personalized medicine approaches in glioblastoma management.

Gene Therapy Approaches in Glioblastoma Treatment

Gene therapy represents a promising strategy for the treatment of glioblastoma, offering the potential to selectively target tumor cells, modulate tumor microenvironment, and overcome treatment resistance through genetic manipulation. In this exploration, we delve into the landscape of gene therapy approaches in glioblastoma treatment, highlighting key strategies, challenges, and future directions in harnessing the power of genetic engineering to combat this aggressive brain tumor.

1. Gene Delivery Systems:

- **Viral Vectors:** Viral vectors, including adenoviruses, lentiviruses, and adeno-associated viruses (AAVs), are commonly used for gene delivery in glioblastoma gene therapy. These vectors offer efficient transduction and stable gene expression in tumor cells, enabling targeted delivery of therapeutic genes and anti-tumor payloads to glioblastoma cells.
- **Non-viral Vectors:** Non-viral vectors, such as liposomes, nanoparticles, and polymer-based carriers, provide alternative gene delivery systems with reduced immunogenicity and safety concerns compared to viral vectors. Non-viral delivery approaches offer flexibility, scalability, and customizable properties for targeted gene therapy applications in glioblastoma.

2. Therapeutic Genes and Strategies:

- **Tumor Suppressor Genes:** Gene therapy approaches targeting tumor suppressor genes, such as p53, PTEN, and RB, aim to restore tumor suppressor function, induce apoptosis, and inhibit tumor growth in glioblastoma. Viral vectors encoding tumor suppressor genes or gene editing technologies, such as CRISPR/Cas9, offer potential strategies to restore tumor suppressor function and enhance therapeutic efficacy.
- **Suicide Genes:** Suicide gene therapy employs prodrug-activating enzymes, such as herpes simplex virus thymidine kinase (HSV-TK) or cytosine deaminase

(CD), which convert non-toxic prodrugs into cytotoxic agents selectively within tumor cells. Suicide gene therapy combined with prodrug administration enables targeted tumor cell killing and bystander effect, resulting in tumor regression and improved survival in glioblastoma models.

- **Immunomodulatory Genes:** Gene therapy approaches targeting immunomodulatory genes, such as cytokines, chemokines, and immune checkpoint inhibitors, aim to modulate the tumor microenvironment, enhance antitumor immune responses, and overcome immunosuppression in glioblastoma. Viral vectors encoding immune stimulatory genes or immune checkpoint inhibitors offer potential strategies to augment antitumor immune responses and improve immunotherapy outcomes in glioblastoma patients.

3. Challenges and Future Directions:

- **Tumor Heterogeneity:** Tumor heterogeneity, characterized by genetic, phenotypic, and spatial diversity within glioblastoma tumors, poses challenges to the efficacy of gene therapy approaches. Strategies to overcome tumor heterogeneity include combination gene therapy approaches targeting multiple pathways, personalized medicine approaches based on molecular profiling, and innovative delivery systems for efficient gene delivery to heterogeneous tumor cell populations.

- **Blood-Brain Barrier (BBB):** The blood-brain barrier (BBB) restricts the delivery of gene therapy vectors and therapeutic agents to the central nervous system (CNS), limiting the efficacy of systemic gene therapy approaches in glioblastoma treatment. Strategies to overcome BBB include local delivery approaches, such as intratumoral injection or convection-enhanced delivery (CED), and BBB disruption techniques, such as focused ultrasound or osmotic agents, to enhance vector penetration into the CNS and improve therapeutic outcomes.

- **Immune Responses:** Immune responses to viral vectors or transgene products may limit the efficacy and safety of gene therapy approaches in glioblastoma treatment. Strategies to mitigate immune responses include vector engineering to reduce immunogenicity, immune modulation strategies to enhance vector persistence and transgene expression, and combination approaches with immunotherapy to augment antitumor immune responses and overcome immune evasion mechanisms.

Conclusion: Gene therapy holds great promise as a novel therapeutic approach for the treatment of glioblastoma, offering targeted and customizable strategies to selectively modulate tumor cells and overcome treatment resistance. By exploring gene delivery systems, therapeutic genes and strategies, and addressing challenges such as tumor heterogeneity, BBB penetration, and immune responses, researchers aim to develop innovative gene therapy approaches with the potential to transform glioblastoma treatment and improve patient outcomes. As the field continues to advance, further refinements in gene therapy techniques, personalized medicine approaches, and combination strategies will be essential for maximizing therapeutic efficacy and translating gene therapy innovations into clinical benefits for glioblastoma patients.

Harnessing Nanotechnology for Glioblastoma Treatment

Nanotechnology offers innovative solutions for addressing the challenges of glioblastoma treatment, including poor drug delivery across the blood-brain barrier, tumor heterogeneity, and treatment resistance. By leveraging the unique properties of nanoparticles, researchers aim to enhance the efficacy, specificity, and safety of therapeutic interventions in glioblastoma. In this exploration, we delve into the application of nanotechnology in glioblastoma treatment, highlighting key strategies, advancements, and future directions in utilizing nanomedicine to combat this aggressive brain tumor.

1. Nanoparticle Formulations:

- **Liposomes:** Liposomes are spherical lipid-based nanoparticles that encapsulate drugs within their lipid bilayer or aqueous core, providing controlled drug release and improved pharmacokinetics. Liposomal formulations offer enhanced drug stability, prolonged circulation time, and selective targeting to glioblastoma cells, enabling efficient drug delivery across the blood-brain barrier and into the tumor microenvironment.

- **Polymeric Nanoparticles:** Polymeric nanoparticles are composed of biocompatible polymers, such as poly(lactic-co-glycolic acid) (PLGA) or polyethylene glycol (PEG), which encapsulate drugs or therapeutic agents for targeted delivery to glioblastoma tumors. Polymeric nanoparticles offer tunable properties, such as size, surface charge, and drug release kinetics, allowing for customizable drug delivery strategies and enhanced tumor penetration.

- **Inorganic Nanoparticles:** Inorganic nanoparticles, including gold nanoparticles, iron oxide nanoparticles, and silica nanoparticles, possess unique physicochemical properties that enable multifunctional applications in glioblastoma therapy. Inorganic nanoparticles can be engineered to deliver drugs, imaging agents, or therapeutic payloads to glioblastoma cells, offering opportunities for combined diagnostics and therapeutics in a single platform.

2. **Targeted Drug Delivery:**
   - **Active Targeting:** Active targeting strategies employ ligands, antibodies, or peptides that selectively bind to receptors or biomarkers overexpressed on glioblastoma cells, facilitating targeted drug delivery and cellular uptake. Targeted nanoparticles can overcome barriers to drug delivery, enhance tumor specificity, and reduce off-target effects, leading to improved therapeutic outcomes and reduced systemic toxicity.
   - **Passive Targeting:** Passive targeting exploits the enhanced permeability and retention (EPR) effect, whereby nanoparticles preferentially accumulate in tumor tissues due to leaky vasculature and impaired lymphatic drainage. Passive targeting enables prolonged circulation time, increased tumor accumulation, and enhanced therapeutic efficacy of nanoparticle-based drugs in glioblastoma treatment.

3. **Therapeutic Applications:**
   - **Chemotherapy:** Nanoparticle-based chemotherapy formulations, such as temozolomide-loaded liposomes or paclitaxel-loaded polymeric nanoparticles, offer improved drug solubility, stability, and tumor targeting in glioblastoma therapy. Nanoparticle-based chemotherapy enables sustained drug release, enhanced tumor penetration, and reduced systemic toxicity compared to conventional chemotherapy agents.
   - **Gene Therapy:** Nanoparticles serve as efficient carriers for delivering nucleic acids, such as siRNA, miRNA, or plasmid DNA, to glioblastoma cells for gene therapy applications. Nanoparticle-mediated gene therapy enables targeted gene delivery, gene silencing, or gene editing in glioblastoma tumors,

offering potential strategies to modulate tumor biology, overcome treatment resistance, and enhance therapeutic efficacy.

4. Imaging and Diagnosis:

- **Magnetic Resonance Imaging (MRI):** Nanoparticles can be functionalized with imaging agents, such as gadolinium chelates or iron oxide nanoparticles, for enhanced contrast in MRI detection of glioblastoma tumors. Nanoparticle-based MRI contrast agents offer improved sensitivity, specificity, and spatial resolution for early detection, accurate diagnosis, and monitoring of glioblastoma progression.

- **Fluorescence Imaging:** Fluorescent nanoparticles, such as quantum dots or organic dyes, enable high-resolution imaging of glioblastoma tumors for intraoperative visualization, image-guided surgery, and real-time monitoring of therapeutic response. Nanoparticle-based fluorescence imaging offers enhanced tumor detection, delineation of tumor margins, and precise localization of residual tumor cells during surgical resection.

5. Challenges and Future Directions:

- **Blood-Brain Barrier Penetration:** Overcoming the blood-brain barrier (BBB) remains a significant challenge for nanoparticle-based drug delivery in glioblastoma treatment. Strategies to enhance BBB penetration include surface modification of nanoparticles, receptor-mediated transcytosis, and temporary disruption of the BBB using focused ultrasound or osmotic agents.

- **Tumor Heterogeneity:** Tumor heterogeneity, characterized by genetic, phenotypic, and spatial diversity within glioblastoma tumors, poses challenges to nanoparticle-based drug delivery and treatment response. Strategies to address tumor heterogeneity include combination nanoparticle formulations targeting multiple pathways, personalized medicine approaches based on molecular profiling, and innovative imaging techniques for real-time monitoring of treatment response.

- **Clinical Translation:** Clinical translation of nanoparticle-based therapies from preclinical studies to human trials requires rigorous evaluation of safety, efficacy, and pharmacokinetics in glioblastoma patients. Multidisciplinary collaborations between researchers, clinicians, and regulatory agencies are essential for advancing nanoparticle-based therapies through clinical development and regulatory approval processes.

Conclusion: Nanotechnology holds tremendous promise for revolutionizing glioblastoma treatment by overcoming the limitations of conventional therapies and enhancing the efficacy, specificity, and safety of therapeutic interventions. By harnessing the unique properties of nanoparticles, researchers aim to develop innovative drug delivery systems, targeted therapies, and imaging agents for precision medicine approaches in glioblastoma therapy. As the field continues to advance, further research into nanoparticle design, optimization, and clinical translation will be essential for realizing the full potential of nanotechnology in improving outcomes for glioblastoma patients.

Exploring Stem Cell Therapy for Glioblastoma Treatment

Stem cell therapy holds promise as a novel approach for the treatment of glioblastoma, leveraging the unique properties of stem cells to target tumor cells, deliver therapeutic agents, and modulate the tumor microenvironment. In this exploration, we delve into the application of stem cell therapy in glioblastoma treatment, highlighting key strategies, advancements, and challenges in harnessing the regenerative potential of stem cells to combat this aggressive brain tumor.

1. Stem Cell Types:
- **Mesenchymal Stem Cells (MSCs):** Mesenchymal stem cells are multipotent adult stem cells with immunomodulatory properties, tropism for tumor sites, and capacity for differentiation into various cell lineages. MSCs offer potential as cellular carriers for targeted delivery of therapeutic agents, such as oncolytic viruses, nanoparticles, or gene therapy vectors, to glioblastoma tumors, enhancing treatment efficacy and reducing off-target effects.
- **Neural Stem Cells (NSCs):** Neural stem cells are self-renewing progenitor cells with the capacity to differentiate into neural lineages, including neurons, astrocytes, and oligodendrocytes. NSCs exhibit tropism for glioblastoma tumors, enabling their preferential migration and integration into tumor sites for targeted delivery of therapeutic payloads, such as cytotoxic agents, tumor-targeting proteins, or RNA interference molecules, to glioblastoma cells.
- **Induced Pluripotent Stem Cells (iPSCs):** Induced pluripotent stem cells are reprogrammed somatic cells with pluripotent properties, capable of differentiating into multiple cell types, including neural progenitor cells and glial cells. iPSC-derived neural progenitor cells offer potential as cellular vehicles for targeted drug delivery, regenerative medicine, and personalized therapy in glioblastoma treatment, providing a scalable and patient-specific approach to treatment.

2. Therapeutic Applications:
- **Targeted Drug Delivery:** Stem cells serve as cellular carriers for targeted delivery of therapeutic agents

to glioblastoma tumors, overcoming barriers to drug delivery, enhancing tumor specificity, and minimizing off-target effects. Stem cell-based drug delivery strategies include encapsulation of drugs within stem cells, surface modification of stem cells with targeting ligands or antibodies, and genetic engineering of stem cells to express therapeutic proteins or RNA interference molecules for targeted therapy.

- **Tumor-Tropic Migration:** Stem cells exhibit tropism for glioblastoma tumors, enabling their preferential migration and homing to tumor sites following systemic or local administration. Tumor-tropic migration of stem cells facilitates their accumulation within glioblastoma tumors, enhancing the specificity and efficacy of stem cell-based therapies, such as targeted drug delivery, tumor imaging, or immunomodulation, in glioblastoma treatment.
- **Immunomodulatory Effects:** Stem cells possess immunomodulatory properties, regulating immune responses, modulating inflammation, and promoting tissue repair in the tumor microenvironment. Stem cell-based immunomodulation strategies aim to harness the immunosuppressive effects of stem cells to inhibit tumor growth, enhance antitumor immune responses, and overcome immunosuppression in glioblastoma, offering potential synergies with conventional therapies, such as chemotherapy, radiation therapy, or immunotherapy.

3. Challenges and Future Directions:

- **Safety Concerns:** Safety concerns, including tumorigenicity, immunogenicity, and off-target effects, remain significant challenges in the clinical translation of stem cell-based therapies for glioblastoma treatment. Strategies to mitigate safety risks include rigorous preclinical evaluation, genetic modification of stem cells for enhanced safety, and monitoring of long-term outcomes in clinical trials to ensure the safety and efficacy of stem cell-based interventions.

- **Optimization of Delivery Strategies:** Optimization of stem cell delivery strategies, including route of administration, timing of delivery, and cell dose, is essential for maximizing the therapeutic efficacy and clinical translation of stem cell-based therapies in glioblastoma treatment. Innovative delivery approaches, such as convection-enhanced delivery (CED), magnetic targeting, or biomaterial scaffolds, offer opportunities to enhance stem cell homing, engraftment, and retention within glioblastoma tumors for targeted therapy.

- **Integration with Standard Therapies:** Integration of stem cell-based therapies with standard treatments, such as surgery, radiation therapy, and chemotherapy, is critical for maximizing treatment efficacy and improving patient outcomes in glioblastoma management. Combination approaches, such as adjuvant stem cell therapy following surgical resection or concurrent stem cell therapy with radiation and chemotherapy, offer potential synergies to enhance tumor control, prolong survival, and improve quality of life for glioblastoma patients.

Conclusion: Stem cell therapy represents a promising approach for the treatment of glioblastoma, harnessing the regenerative potential of stem cells to target tumor cells, deliver therapeutic agents, and modulate the tumor microenvironment. By exploring different stem cell types, therapeutic applications, and addressing challenges such as safety concerns, delivery optimization, and integration with standard therapies, researchers aim to develop innovative stem cell-based treatments that offer improved efficacy, reduced toxicity, and enhanced patient outcomes in the management of this aggressive brain tumor. As the field continues to advance, further research into stem cell biology, preclinical models, and clinical trials will be essential for realizing the full potential of stem cell therapy in glioblastoma treatment and translating stem cell-based innovations into clinical benefits for patients.

Immunomodulatory Strategies in Glioblastoma Therapy: Unleashing the Power of the Immune System

Glioblastoma, a highly aggressive brain tumor, poses significant therapeutic challenges due to its ability to evade immune surveillance and suppress antitumor immune responses. Immunomodulatory strategies aim to harness the innate and adaptive immune systems to recognize and eliminate glioblastoma cells, offering potential avenues for enhancing treatment efficacy and improving patient outcomes. In this exploration, we delve into the landscape of immunomodulatory strategies in glioblastoma therapy, highlighting key mechanisms, therapeutic approaches, and challenges in harnessing the power of the immune system to combat this devastating disease.

1. **Immune Evasion Mechanisms in Glioblastoma:** Glioblastoma employs multiple strategies to evade immune detection and suppress antitumor immune responses, including:
    - **Immune Checkpoint Signaling:** Glioblastoma cells upregulate immune checkpoint molecules, such as programmed cell death protein 1 (PD-1), programmed death-ligand 1 (PD-L1), and cytotoxic T-lymphocyte-associated protein 4 (CTLA-4), to inhibit T cell activation and promote immune evasion.
    - **Tumor-Mediated Immunosuppression:** Glioblastoma creates an immunosuppressive microenvironment through the secretion of immunosuppressive

cytokines, recruitment of regulatory T cells (Tregs) and myeloid-derived suppressor cells (MDSCs), and expression of inhibitory ligands on tumor cells and immune cells.

2. Immunotherapy Approaches: Immunotherapy represents a promising approach for overcoming immune evasion and enhancing antitumor immune responses in glioblastoma, including:

- **Checkpoint Inhibitors:** Checkpoint inhibitors, such as anti-PD-1 antibodies (e.g., pembrolizumab, nivolumab) and anti-PD-L1 antibodies (e.g., atezolizumab, durvalumab), block immune checkpoint signaling pathways, releasing the brakes on T cell activation and restoring antitumor immune responses.
- **Vaccines:** Therapeutic vaccines, such as dendritic cell vaccines, peptide vaccines, and tumor cell vaccines, stimulate the immune system to recognize and target glioblastoma-specific antigens, inducing antitumor immune responses and immunological memory.
- **CAR-T Cell Therapy:** Chimeric antigen receptor (CAR) T cell therapy involves engineering patients' T cells to express CARs targeting glioblastoma-associated antigens, such as EGFRvIII or IL13Rα2, enabling targeted tumor cell recognition and destruction by engineered T cells.

3. Combination Therapies: Combination approaches, including immunotherapy in combination with standard treatments or other immunomodulatory agents, hold promise for enhancing treatment efficacy and overcoming resistance mechanisms in glioblastoma, such as:

- **Radiotherapy and Chemotherapy:** Radiotherapy and chemotherapy can modulate the tumor microenvironment, enhance tumor antigen presentation, and sensitize glioblastoma cells

to immune-mediated killing, synergizing with immunotherapy to improve treatment outcomes.
- **Targeted Therapies:** Targeted therapies, such as EGFR inhibitors (e.g., erlotinib, gefitinib) or angiogenesis inhibitors (e.g., bevacizumab), may enhance immunotherapy responses by reducing tumor burden, normalizing the tumor vasculature, and modulating immune cell trafficking and infiltration in glioblastoma tumors.

4. Challenges and Future Directions: Despite the promise of immunomodulatory strategies in glioblastoma therapy, several challenges remain to be addressed, including:
- **Tumor Heterogeneity:** Glioblastoma exhibits extensive intratumoral and intertumoral heterogeneity, posing challenges for immunotherapy efficacy and response prediction. Strategies to overcome tumor heterogeneity include combination immunotherapy approaches targeting multiple pathways and personalized medicine approaches based on molecular profiling.
- **Blood-Brain Barrier (BBB):** The blood-brain barrier (BBB) restricts the penetration of immune cells and therapeutic agents into the central nervous system (CNS), limiting the efficacy of immunomodulatory strategies in glioblastoma treatment. Strategies to overcome BBB include local delivery approaches, such as convection-enhanced delivery (CED), and BBB disruption techniques, such as focused ultrasound or osmotic agents, to enhance immune cell trafficking and infiltration into the CNS.
- **Resistance Mechanisms:** Glioblastoma cells may develop resistance to immunotherapy through various mechanisms, including upregulation of alternative immune checkpoints, loss of tumor antigens, and recruitment of immunosuppressive cells. Strategies

to overcome resistance include combination immunotherapy approaches, rational design of CAR constructs, and identification of predictive biomarkers to guide treatment selection and monitoring.

Conclusion: Immunomodulatory strategies offer promising avenues for enhancing treatment efficacy and improving outcomes in glioblastoma therapy by harnessing the power of the immune system to recognize and eliminate tumor cells. By exploring checkpoint inhibitors, vaccines, CAR-T cell therapy, and combination approaches, researchers aim to overcome immune evasion mechanisms, enhance antitumor immune responses, and overcome resistance mechanisms in glioblastoma treatment. As the field continues to advance, further research into tumor immunology, biomarker discovery, and clinical trial design will be essential for translating immunomodulatory innovations into effective therapies for glioblastoma patients, ultimately improving survival and quality of life for those affected by this devastating disease.

Precision Medicine and Personalized Treatment in Glioblastoma: Tailoring Therapy to the Individual

Glioblastoma, characterized by its heterogeneity and aggressive nature, necessitates a personalized approach to treatment that accounts for the unique molecular and genetic characteristics of each patient's tumor. Precision medicine offers the opportunity to tailor therapy based on specific biomarkers, genetic alterations, and molecular subtypes, thereby optimizing treatment outcomes and minimizing adverse effects. In this exploration, we delve into the principles of precision medicine and personalized treatment in glioblastoma, highlighting key strategies, advancements, and challenges in delivering targeted therapies to individual patients.

1. Molecular Profiling and Biomarker Identification: Molecular profiling of glioblastoma tumors enables the identification of specific biomarkers, genetic alterations, and molecular subtypes that inform treatment selection and prognostic assessment, including:

- **Genomic Alterations:** Genetic alterations, such as mutations in the IDH1/2 genes, EGFR amplification, PTEN loss, and MGMT promoter methylation status, serve as prognostic and predictive biomarkers in glioblastoma, guiding treatment decisions and predicting treatment response.
- **Molecular Subtypes:** Glioblastoma tumors can be classified into distinct molecular subtypes, such as classical, mesenchymal, proneural, and neural subtypes, based on gene expression profiles and molecular signatures, which have implications for treatment response and patient outcomes.

2. Targeted Therapies and Personalized Treatment Strategies: Targeted therapies aim to exploit specific molecular vulnerabilities and pathways in glioblastoma tumors, offering personalized treatment options tailored to individual patients, including:

- **EGFR Inhibitors:** EGFR inhibitors, such as erlotinib, gefitinib, and lapatinib, target the epidermal growth factor receptor (EGFR) pathway, which is frequently dysregulated in glioblastoma tumors with EGFR amplification or mutation, offering potential therapeutic benefits in selected patients.
- **PI3K/mTOR Inhibitors:** Inhibitors of the phosphatidylinositol 3-kinase (PI3K) and mammalian target of rapamycin (mTOR) pathways, such as temsirolimus, everolimus, and sirolimus, target downstream signaling pathways activated in glioblastoma tumors with PTEN loss or PI3K pathway alterations, providing personalized treatment options for patients with specific molecular profiles.

- **IDH Inhibitors:** IDH inhibitors, such as ivosidenib and enasidenib, target mutant isocitrate dehydrogenase (IDH) enzymes, which are prevalent in glioblastoma tumors with IDH1/2 mutations, offering personalized treatment options for patients with IDH-mutant tumors.

3. Combination Therapies and Adaptive Treatment Strategies: Combination therapies combine targeted agents with conventional treatments, such as surgery, radiation therapy, and chemotherapy, to enhance treatment efficacy and overcome resistance mechanisms in glioblastoma tumors, including:

- **Radiotherapy and Chemotherapy:** Radiation therapy and chemotherapy, such as temozolomide, can modulate the tumor microenvironment, sensitize glioblastoma cells to targeted therapies, and enhance treatment responses in combination with targeted agents.
- **Immunotherapy and Targeted Therapy:** Immunotherapy approaches, such as checkpoint inhibitors or CAR-T cell therapy, can be combined with targeted therapies to enhance antitumor immune responses, overcome immune evasion mechanisms, and improve treatment outcomes in glioblastoma patients.

4. Challenges and Future Directions: Despite the promise of precision medicine and personalized treatment in glioblastoma therapy, several challenges remain to be addressed, including:

- **Biomarker Validation:** Validation of biomarkers and molecular subtypes in large-scale clinical trials is essential for establishing their clinical utility and predictive value in guiding treatment decisions and optimizing patient outcomes.
- **Resistance Mechanisms:** Glioblastoma tumors may develop resistance to targeted therapies through

various mechanisms, including activation of alternative signaling pathways, adaptive immune responses, and clonal evolution. Strategies to overcome resistance include combination therapies, adaptive treatment strategies, and identification of novel therapeutic targets.

- **Clinical Implementation:** Integration of precision medicine approaches into routine clinical practice requires multidisciplinary collaboration, infrastructure support, and evidence-based guidelines for biomarker testing, treatment selection, and patient management in glioblastoma therapy.

Conclusion: Precision medicine and personalized treatment offer a transformative approach to glioblastoma therapy, tailoring treatment to the individual characteristics of each patient's tumor and optimizing therapeutic outcomes. By leveraging molecular profiling, targeted therapies, combination approaches, and adaptive treatment strategies, researchers aim to overcome treatment resistance, improve survival, and enhance quality of life for glioblastoma patients. As the field continues to advance, further research into biomarker discovery, clinical validation, and implementation strategies will be essential for realizing the full potential of precision medicine in transforming glioblastoma treatment and improving patient outcomes.

CHAPTER 9: SUPPORTIVE CARE AND HOLISTIC APPROACHES

Nutritional Support in Glioblastoma Therapy: Nourishing the Body, Nurturing the Soul

Nutritional support plays a crucial role in the holistic care of glioblastoma patients, providing essential nutrients, managing treatment-related side effects, and optimizing overall health and well-being throughout the disease journey. In this exploration, we delve into the importance of nutritional support in glioblastoma therapy, highlighting key considerations, dietary strategies, and supportive interventions aimed at nourishing the body and nurturing the soul of patients facing this challenging diagnosis.

1. Nutritional Challenges in Glioblastoma: Glioblastoma and its treatments pose significant challenges to nutritional status and metabolic health, including:

- **Cachexia:** Glioblastoma patients are at risk of developing cachexia, a complex metabolic syndrome characterized by involuntary weight loss, muscle wasting, and systemic inflammation, which negatively impacts quality of life, treatment tolerance, and survival outcomes.

- **Treatment-Related Side Effects:** Surgery, radiation therapy, and chemotherapy can induce a range of treatment-related side effects, such as nausea, vomiting, dysphagia, taste changes, and fatigue, which may affect appetite, nutrient intake, and nutritional status in glioblastoma patients.

2. **Nutritional Goals and Considerations:** Nutritional support in glioblastoma therapy aims to achieve several goals, including:

- **Optimizing Nutrient Intake:** Ensuring adequate intake of essential nutrients, such as protein, vitamins, minerals, and antioxidants, to support immune function, tissue repair, and overall health in glioblastoma patients.
- **Managing Treatment Side Effects:** Addressing treatment-related side effects, such as nausea, vomiting, dysphagia, and taste changes, through dietary modifications, symptom management strategies, and supportive interventions to improve nutritional status and quality of life.
- **Preventing Malnutrition:** Preventing or mitigating malnutrition, cachexia, and sarcopenia through early nutritional intervention, personalized dietary counseling, and supportive care measures to optimize treatment outcomes and patient well-being.

3. **Dietary Strategies and Nutritional Interventions:** Dietary strategies and nutritional interventions play a critical role in supporting glioblastoma patients throughout their treatment journey, including:

- **Individualized Meal Planning:** Tailoring meal plans to meet the specific nutritional needs, preferences, and tolerances of glioblastoma patients, considering factors such as caloric requirements, macronutrient distribution, and dietary restrictions.
- **High-Calorie, High-Protein Foods:** Incorporating

nutrient-dense foods, such as lean proteins, whole grains, fruits, vegetables, and healthy fats, into the diet to provide essential nutrients and promote energy intake and muscle preservation in glioblastoma patients.

- **Supplemental Nutrition:** Providing oral nutritional supplements, enteral nutrition support, or parenteral nutrition as needed to supplement caloric intake, manage treatment-related side effects, and prevent malnutrition in glioblastoma patients unable to meet their nutritional needs through oral intake alone.

4. Supportive Care and Holistic Approaches: In addition to dietary strategies, supportive care and holistic approaches are integral components of nutritional support in glioblastoma therapy, including:

- **Symptom Management:** Addressing treatment-related side effects, such as nausea, vomiting, dysphagia, and taste changes, through pharmacological interventions, dietary modifications, and complementary therapies to improve symptom control and enhance quality of life.
- **Psychosocial Support:** Providing psychosocial support, counseling, and resources to glioblastoma patients and their families to cope with the emotional, psychological, and social challenges of the disease, promote mental well-being, and foster resilience throughout the treatment journey.
- **Physical Activity and Rehabilitation:** Incorporating physical activity, rehabilitation exercises, and supportive therapies, such as physical therapy, occupational therapy, and speech therapy, into the care plan to optimize functional capacity, mobility, and independence in glioblastoma patients.

5. Challenges and Future Directions: Despite the importance of nutritional support in glioblastoma therapy, several challenges remain to be addressed, including:

- **Patient Adherence:** Ensuring patient adherence to dietary recommendations, nutritional interventions, and supportive care measures throughout the treatment journey, particularly in the face of treatment-related side effects, appetite changes, and psychosocial stressors.
- **Multidisciplinary Collaboration:** Facilitating multidisciplinary collaboration among healthcare providers, including oncologists, dietitians, nurses, and allied health professionals, to coordinate nutritional support, symptom management, and supportive care interventions for glioblastoma patients.
- **Research and Innovation:** Advancing research and innovation in the field of nutritional oncology, including clinical trials, evidence-based guidelines, and novel interventions, to optimize nutritional support, improve treatment outcomes, and enhance quality of life for glioblastoma patients.

Conclusion: Nutritional support is an essential component of holistic care in glioblastoma therapy, providing vital nourishment, managing treatment-related side effects, and optimizing overall health and well-being throughout the disease journey. By addressing nutritional challenges, implementing dietary strategies, and incorporating supportive care measures, healthcare providers can support glioblastoma patients in maintaining optimal nutritional status, enhancing treatment tolerance, and improving quality of life. As the field continues to evolve, further research, education, and collaboration will be essential for advancing nutritional support in glioblastoma therapy and delivering personalized care to patients facing this challenging diagnosis.

Physical Rehabilitation in Glioblastoma Therapy: Restoring Function, Enhancing Quality of Life

Physical rehabilitation plays a crucial role in the comprehensive care of glioblastoma patients, focusing on restoring physical function, improving mobility, and enhancing quality of life throughout the treatment journey. In this exploration, we delve into the importance of physical rehabilitation in glioblastoma therapy, highlighting key principles, therapeutic modalities, and supportive interventions aimed at optimizing functional outcomes and promoting well-being for patients facing this challenging diagnosis.

1. Functional Impairments in Glioblastoma: Glioblastoma and its treatments can lead to a range of physical impairments and functional limitations, including:

- **Motor Deficits:** Glioblastoma tumors located in motor areas of the brain can result in weakness, paralysis, and coordination difficulties, affecting mobility and activities of daily living (ADLs).
- **Balance and Coordination:** Glioblastoma patients may experience balance disturbances, dizziness, and coordination problems due to disruptions in sensorimotor pathways, increasing the risk of falls and mobility limitations.
- **Cognitive and Perceptual Changes:** Glioblastoma-associated cognitive deficits, such as memory impairment, attentional deficits, and executive dysfunction, can impact participation in rehabilitation activities and ADLs.

2. Goals of Physical Rehabilitation: Physical rehabilitation in glioblastoma therapy aims to achieve several key goals, including:

- **Restoring Physical Function:** Restoring mobility,

strength, flexibility, and endurance to maximize functional independence and quality of life for glioblastoma patients.
- **Improving Motor Control:** Enhancing motor control, coordination, and balance to facilitate safe and efficient movement patterns and reduce the risk of falls and injuries.
- **Enhancing Quality of Life:** Improving overall well-being, psychological adjustment, and social participation through physical activity, exercise, and supportive interventions.

3. Therapeutic Modalities and Rehabilitation Strategies: Physical rehabilitation employs a variety of therapeutic modalities and rehabilitation strategies tailored to the individual needs and goals of glioblastoma patients, including:
- **Exercise Therapy:** Structured exercise programs, including aerobic conditioning, strength training, flexibility exercises, and balance training, help improve physical fitness, functional capacity, and overall well-being in glioblastoma patients.
- **Gait Training:** Gait training exercises, such as treadmill walking, overground walking, and stair climbing, focus on improving walking ability, balance, and coordination in glioblastoma patients with mobility impairments.
- **Neuromuscular Reeducation:** Neuromuscular reeducation techniques, including proprioceptive exercises, mirror therapy, and task-specific training, aim to enhance motor control, coordination, and movement patterns in glioblastoma patients with sensorimotor deficits.
- **Assistive Devices:** Assistive devices, such as canes, walkers, orthoses, and mobility aids, provide support and assistance to glioblastoma patients with

mobility limitations, facilitating safe and independent movement.

4. Multidisciplinary Approach and Collaborative Care: Physical rehabilitation in glioblastoma therapy requires a multidisciplinary approach and collaborative care among healthcare providers, including:

- **Rehabilitation Team:** A multidisciplinary rehabilitation team, including physical therapists, occupational therapists, speech therapists, and rehabilitation nurses, collaborates to assess functional impairments, develop individualized treatment plans, and monitor progress throughout the rehabilitation process.
- **Oncology Team:** Close coordination with the oncology team, including neurosurgeons, radiation oncologists, medical oncologists, and palliative care specialists, ensures comprehensive care and integration of rehabilitation into the overall treatment plan for glioblastoma patients.

5. Challenges and Future Directions: Despite the importance of physical rehabilitation in glioblastoma therapy, several challenges remain to be addressed, including:

- **Functional Limitations:** Severe functional impairments, cognitive deficits, and communication difficulties may present challenges to participation in rehabilitation activities and achieving functional goals in glioblastoma patients.
- **Treatment-Related Fatigue:** Treatment-related fatigue, weakness, and deconditioning can impact motivation, adherence, and progress in physical rehabilitation programs, requiring tailored interventions and supportive strategies to address fatigue management and energy conservation.
- **Psychosocial Support:** Psychosocial factors, including

emotional distress, depression, anxiety, and caregiver burden, may influence engagement, adherence, and outcomes in physical rehabilitation, highlighting the importance of psychosocial support services and holistic care approaches for glioblastoma patients and their families.

Conclusion: Physical rehabilitation plays a vital role in the comprehensive care of glioblastoma patients, focusing on restoring physical function, improving mobility, and enhancing quality of life throughout the treatment journey. By addressing functional impairments, implementing therapeutic modalities, and fostering collaborative care, physical rehabilitation aims to optimize functional outcomes, promote well-being, and empower glioblastoma patients to live life to the fullest despite the challenges they face. As the field continues to evolve, further research, innovation, and multidisciplinary collaboration will be essential for advancing physical rehabilitation in glioblastoma therapy and improving outcomes for patients affected by this devastating disease.

Psychosocial Support and Counseling in Glioblastoma Therapy: Nurturing the Mind, Strengthening the Spirit

Glioblastoma, a diagnosis fraught with uncertainty and emotional turmoil, not only impacts the physical health of patients but also profoundly affects their psychological well-being and quality of life. Psychosocial support and counseling play a pivotal role in the holistic care of glioblastoma patients, providing emotional support, coping strategies, and resilience-building interventions to navigate the challenges of the disease journey. In this exploration, we delve into the importance of psychosocial support and counseling in glioblastoma therapy, highlighting key principles, therapeutic approaches, and supportive interventions aimed at nurturing the mind and strengthening the spirit of patients facing this formidable diagnosis.

1. Psychological Impact of Glioblastoma: Glioblastoma poses significant psychological challenges and emotional distress for patients and their families, including:

- **Fear and Uncertainty:** The diagnosis of glioblastoma often evokes fear, uncertainty, and existential distress, as patients confront the reality of a life-threatening illness and uncertain prognosis.
- **Anxiety and Depression:** Glioblastoma patients may experience heightened levels of anxiety, depression, and psychological distress due to the stress of diagnosis, treatment-related side effects, and concerns about the future.
- **Loss and Grief:** Glioblastoma patients and their families may experience profound feelings of loss, grief, and mourning as they confront changes in physical function, cognitive abilities, and quality of life associated with the disease.

2. Goals of Psychosocial Support and Counseling: Psychosocial support and counseling in glioblastoma therapy aim to achieve several key goals, including:

- **Emotional Support:** Providing empathic listening, validation, and emotional support to glioblastoma patients and their families, acknowledging their fears, concerns, and coping strategies.
- **Coping Strategies:** Equipping patients and caregivers with coping strategies, resilience-building techniques, and problem-solving skills to navigate the challenges of the disease journey and promote adaptive coping.
- **Quality of Life:** Enhancing overall well-being, psychological adjustment, and quality of life for glioblastoma patients and their families through psychosocial interventions, supportive care, and holistic approaches.

3. Therapeutic Approaches and Supportive Interventions: Psychosocial support and counseling encompass a range of therapeutic approaches and supportive interventions tailored to the individual needs and preferences of glioblastoma patients and their families, including:

- **Individual Counseling:** One-on-one counseling sessions with a trained psychologist, social worker, or counselor provide a safe and supportive space for patients to explore their thoughts, feelings, and concerns, process grief and loss, and develop coping strategies for managing distress.
- **Family Therapy:** Family therapy sessions involve patients and their family members in collaborative discussions, communication exercises, and problem-solving techniques to enhance family cohesion, support networks, and coping skills in the face of glioblastoma diagnosis and treatment.
- **Support Groups:** Peer support groups, facilitated by trained professionals or led by fellow patients and caregivers, offer opportunities for shared experiences, mutual support, and coping strategies among individuals affected by glioblastoma, fostering a sense of community and belonging.
- **Mind-Body Interventions:** Mind-body interventions, such as mindfulness meditation, relaxation techniques, guided imagery, and yoga, promote stress reduction, emotional regulation, and psychological well-being in glioblastoma patients and their caregivers.

4. Multidisciplinary Collaboration and Holistic Care: Psychosocial support and counseling in glioblastoma therapy require a multidisciplinary approach and collaborative care among healthcare providers, including:

- **Oncology Team:** Close collaboration with the oncology

team, including neurosurgeons, radiation oncologists, medical oncologists, and palliative care specialists, ensures comprehensive care and integration of psychosocial support into the overall treatment plan for glioblastoma patients.
- **Rehabilitation Team:** Coordination with the rehabilitation team, including physical therapists, occupational therapists, speech therapists, and rehabilitation nurses, addresses functional impairments, cognitive deficits, and psychosocial challenges in glioblastoma patients throughout the treatment journey.

5. Challenges and Future Directions: Despite the importance of psychosocial support and counseling in glioblastoma therapy, several challenges remain to be addressed, including:
- **Access and Equity:** Ensuring equitable access to psychosocial support services, counseling resources, and supportive interventions for all glioblastoma patients and their families, regardless of socioeconomic status, geographical location, or healthcare setting.
- **Stigma and Mental Health:** Addressing stigma, misconceptions, and barriers to seeking mental health support and counseling among glioblastoma patients and their families, promoting destigmatization, awareness, and acceptance of psychological well-being as integral to holistic care.
- **Research and Innovation:** Advancing research and innovation in the field of psycho-oncology, including clinical trials, evidence-based interventions, and novel approaches to psychosocial support and counseling, to optimize outcomes, improve access, and enhance quality of life for glioblastoma patients and their families.

Conclusion: Psychosocial support and counseling play a vital role in the holistic care of glioblastoma patients, providing emotional support, coping strategies, and resilience-building interventions to navigate the challenges of the disease journey. By addressing psychological distress, promoting adaptive coping, and fostering a sense of community and belonging, psychosocial support aims to nurture the mind and strengthen the spirit of patients facing this formidable diagnosis. As the field continues to evolve, further research, education, and collaboration will be essential for advancing psychosocial support and counseling in glioblastoma therapy and improving outcomes for patients and their families affected by this devastating disease.

Integrative Medicine in Glioblastoma Therapy: Harmonizing Body, Mind, and Spirit

Integrative medicine offers a holistic approach to care in glioblastoma therapy, encompassing conventional treatments alongside complementary and alternative therapies aimed at promoting healing, enhancing well-being, and optimizing quality of life for patients facing this formidable diagnosis. In this exploration, we delve into the principles of integrative medicine in glioblastoma therapy, highlighting key modalities, therapeutic approaches, and supportive interventions aimed at harmonizing body, mind, and spirit to support patients on their journey toward healing and wholeness.

1. **Principles of Integrative Medicine:** Integrative medicine embraces a patient-centered approach to care, emphasizing the following principles:
    - **Whole-Person Care:** Recognizing the interconnectedness of body, mind, and spirit and addressing the physical, emotional, social, and spiritual dimensions of health and well-being in glioblastoma patients.

- **Patient Empowerment:** Empowering patients to actively participate in their healing journey, make informed decisions about their care, and engage in self-care practices that promote resilience and well-being.
- **Collaborative Care:** Fostering collaboration among healthcare providers, including conventional oncologists, integrative medicine practitioners, and allied health professionals, to provide comprehensive, coordinated care tailored to the individual needs and preferences of glioblastoma patients.

2. Therapeutic Modalities in Integrative Medicine: Integrative medicine incorporates a variety of therapeutic modalities and healing practices aimed at supporting the body's innate capacity for healing and promoting holistic well-being, including:

- **Acupuncture:** Acupuncture, an ancient Chinese healing art, involves the insertion of thin needles into specific acupoints on the body to restore the flow of qi (vital energy) and balance the body's energy systems, offering pain relief, stress reduction, and relaxation for glioblastoma patients.
- **Meditation and Mindfulness:** Meditation and mindfulness practices cultivate present-moment awareness, attentional focus, and emotional regulation, reducing stress, anxiety, and psychological distress in glioblastoma patients and promoting a sense of inner peace and resilience.
- **Yoga and Tai Chi:** Yoga and tai chi combine movement, breathwork, and mindfulness practices to promote physical fitness, flexibility, and relaxation, enhancing overall well-being and quality of life for glioblastoma patients.
- **Nutritional Counseling:** Nutritional counseling provides personalized dietary guidance, nutrition

education, and lifestyle recommendations to optimize nutrition, support immune function, and mitigate treatment-related side effects in glioblastoma patients.
- **Herbal Medicine and Supplements:** Herbal medicine and dietary supplements, such as herbs, vitamins, minerals, and botanical extracts, offer supportive interventions to complement conventional treatments, alleviate symptoms, and promote healing in glioblastoma patients.

3. Supportive Care and Holistic Approaches: Integrative medicine emphasizes supportive care and holistic approaches to healing, including:
- **Pain Management:** Integrative pain management approaches, such as acupuncture, massage therapy, and mind-body techniques, offer non-pharmacological options for pain relief and symptom management in glioblastoma patients, minimizing reliance on opioid medications and their associated side effects.
- **Stress Reduction:** Stress reduction techniques, such as relaxation exercises, guided imagery, and biofeedback, help glioblastoma patients cope with the emotional and psychological challenges of the disease journey, promoting emotional resilience and well-being.
- **Spiritual Care:** Spiritual care interventions, such as prayer, meditation, and pastoral counseling, address the existential and spiritual concerns of glioblastoma patients, providing comfort, meaning, and support in times of uncertainty and distress.

4. Challenges and Future Directions: Despite the potential benefits of integrative medicine in glioblastoma therapy, several challenges remain to be addressed, including:
- **Evidence Base:** Limited scientific evidence and research on the efficacy and safety of integrative medicine interventions in glioblastoma therapy,

highlighting the need for rigorous clinical trials, outcome studies, and evidence-based guidelines to inform clinical practice and decision-making.

- **Integration into Conventional Care:** Integration of integrative medicine approaches into conventional oncology settings, including collaborative care models, interdisciplinary communication, and provider education, to ensure safe, effective, and coordinated care for glioblastoma patients.
- **Access and Equity:** Access to integrative medicine services, resources, and supportive interventions for all glioblastoma patients, regardless of socioeconomic status, geographical location, or healthcare setting, to promote equity, inclusion, and patient-centered care.

Conclusion: Integrative medicine offers a holistic approach to care in glioblastoma therapy, integrating conventional treatments with complementary and alternative therapies aimed at promoting healing, enhancing well-being, and optimizing quality of life for patients facing this formidable diagnosis. By embracing whole-person care, empowering patients, fostering collaborative care, and promoting supportive interventions, integrative medicine seeks to harmonize body, mind, and spirit and support patients on their journey toward healing and wholeness. As the field continues to evolve, further research, education, and collaboration will be essential for advancing integrative medicine in glioblastoma therapy and improving outcomes for patients affected by this devastating disease.

Lifestyle Modifications for Cancer Prevention and Management: Empowering Health Beyond Treatment

In the fight against cancer, lifestyle modifications play a pivotal role in prevention, management, and survivorship, offering patients and survivors the opportunity to take an active role in their health and well-being. Glioblastoma patients, in particular, can benefit from adopting healthy lifestyle practices that support overall health, enhance treatment outcomes, and improve quality of life. In this exploration, we delve into the importance of lifestyle modifications for cancer prevention and management, highlighting key strategies, behaviors, and habits aimed at empowering health beyond treatment for glioblastoma patients and survivors.

1. Importance of Lifestyle Modifications: Lifestyle modifications offer numerous benefits for cancer prevention, management, and survivorship, including:

- **Reduced Risk:** Adopting healthy lifestyle practices, such as maintaining a balanced diet, engaging in regular physical activity, avoiding tobacco and excessive alcohol consumption, and managing stress, can reduce the risk of developing cancer and other chronic diseases.
- **Enhanced Treatment Outcomes:** Lifestyle modifications, such as nutrition optimization, exercise promotion, and stress reduction, can enhance treatment tolerance, support immune function, and improve treatment outcomes for cancer patients undergoing surgery, radiation therapy, and chemotherapy.
- **Improved Quality of Life:** Lifestyle modifications contribute to overall well-being, psychological adjustment, and quality of life for cancer survivors, promoting physical fitness, emotional resilience, and social connectedness beyond the cancer diagnosis and treatment journey.

2. Key Lifestyle Modifications for Glioblastoma Patients: Glioblastoma patients can benefit from adopting the following lifestyle modifications to support their health and well-being:

- **Healthy Eating:** Emphasize a balanced diet rich in

fruits, vegetables, whole grains, lean proteins, and healthy fats to provide essential nutrients, support immune function, and optimize overall health and well-being.
- **Regular Exercise:** Engage in regular physical activity, such as walking, swimming, cycling, or yoga, to improve physical fitness, enhance mobility, and reduce fatigue during and after treatment for glioblastoma.
- **Tobacco Cessation:** Avoid tobacco use and exposure to secondhand smoke, as smoking is associated with an increased risk of cancer recurrence, treatment complications, and other health issues for glioblastoma patients.
- **Alcohol Moderation:** Limit alcohol consumption to moderate levels, as excessive alcohol intake is linked to an increased risk of cancer development, treatment-related side effects, and other health problems in glioblastoma patients.
- **Stress Management:** Practice stress reduction techniques, such as mindfulness meditation, deep breathing exercises, progressive muscle relaxation, or guided imagery, to reduce stress, anxiety, and psychological distress associated with glioblastoma diagnosis and treatment.

3. Supportive Resources and Services: Glioblastoma patients can access a variety of supportive resources and services to facilitate lifestyle modifications and promote overall health and well-being, including:
- **Nutrition Counseling:** Consult with a registered dietitian or nutritionist for personalized nutrition guidance, dietary recommendations, and meal planning strategies to support optimal nutrition during and after treatment for glioblastoma.
- **Exercise Programs:** Participate in structured exercise

programs, rehabilitation therapies, or physical activity classes tailored to the individual needs and preferences of glioblastoma patients, promoting physical fitness, functional capacity, and overall well-being.

- **Smoking Cessation Programs:** Enroll in smoking cessation programs, support groups, or counseling services to quit smoking, reduce tobacco use, and improve lung health for glioblastoma patients and survivors.
- **Stress Reduction Workshops:** Attend stress reduction workshops, relaxation classes, or mindfulness-based programs to learn effective stress management techniques, coping strategies, and resilience-building skills for navigating the challenges of glioblastoma diagnosis and treatment.

4. Empowerment and Self-Care: Empowering glioblastoma patients to take an active role in their health and well-being through lifestyle modifications and self-care practices is essential for promoting resilience, fostering a sense of control, and enhancing quality of life beyond treatment. By embracing healthy habits, seeking supportive resources, and cultivating a positive mindset, glioblastoma patients can optimize their overall health and well-being and empower themselves to thrive in the face of adversity.

Conclusion: Lifestyle modifications offer glioblastoma patients and survivors the opportunity to take control of their health and well-being, reduce the risk of cancer recurrence, enhance treatment outcomes, and improve quality of life beyond the cancer diagnosis and treatment journey. By adopting healthy eating habits, engaging in regular physical activity, avoiding tobacco and excessive alcohol consumption, and practicing stress management techniques, glioblastoma patients can empower themselves to lead healthier, happier lives and optimize their overall health and well-being. As the field of oncology continues to evolve, further research, education, and advocacy will be essential for promoting lifestyle modifications as integral components of cancer prevention, management, and survivorship care for glioblastoma patients and survivors.

Printed in Great Britain
by Amazon